Gout Recipes

Anti – Inflammatory Natural Food Ingredients

Peter Voit

Hi, I am Peter. And I have been dealing with Gout for several years now. I have learned to control it through my diet, and regular exercise. I want to share with you some of my favorite recipes, that I use on a regular basis. Always consult with your Doctors if you are adding any foods into your diet. As every person is unique as to what we can, and cannot eat. I tend to eat more of a plant based diet for the most part. I do eat meat occasionally. And personally can have most seafoods. These recipes are mostly plant based. With some containing eggs, and options for a little dairy. Always substitute ingredients that you may not eat. Enjoy these recipes!
Peter

Table of Contents

Tofu Basil Eggplant 42

Veggie Pita Pockets 45

Gout Friendly Pizza 47

Baked Tofu and Roasted Peppers 49

Eggplant Chickpea 51

Kale and Tofu 53

Stuffed Pepper Melts 55

Marinated Mint Eggplant 57

Spiced Eggplant 59

Eggplant with Quinoa 62

Red Potato Mix 64

Potato Spinach Casserole 67

Mushroom Kabobs 70

Garbanzo Curry 72

Ginger Stir-Fry with Coconut Rice 75

Lime – Strawberry - Spinach Smoothie 79

Lime - Honeydew Smoothie 82

Orange - Peach - Raspberry Smoothie 84

Vanilla - Cinnamon Smoothie 87

Minty Pineapple Smoothie 89

Mango Madness Smoothie 91

Cherry Berry Smoothie 93

Green Goodness Smoothie 95

Join the free Gout & Inflammation Newsletter.
Clickable links are inside of the eBook version
of this book. Or, you can also email
goutinflammationinfo@gmail.com
and request the link to be sent to your email.

Ginger Sweet Potato Soup

Ingredients:

- 1 tablespoon olive oil
- 2 medium-large sweet potatoes peeled, chopped, and pureed
- 1 clove garlic
- ½ inch grated ginger
- 1 teaspoon turmeric
- 4 diced mint leaves
- 2 cup no sodium vegetable broth

Directions:

1. Pour olive oil into food processor
2. Wash, peel, cut into small pieces, and place sweet potato bits into the food processor with the oil.
3. Add garlic clove to the food processor
4. Add the ginger, turmeric.
5. Wash, dry, and chop mint leaves.
6. Puree
7. Pour into medium sized pot or Dutch oven
8. Add broth
9. Let sit over medium-medium high heat 25-30 minutes.
10. Serve as a side, or main dish.

Nutritional Info:
Calories: 240
Total Fats: 4 g
Carbohydrates: 46 g
Protein: 4g

RECIPE

Sweet Avocado Cabbage Rolls

Ingredients:

- 1 tablespoon extra virgin coconut oil
- 1 – 2 tablespoons apple cider vinegar
- 1 large avocado diced
- 1 head of green cabbage
- 1 small sweet onion diced
- ½ tablespoon cayenne powder

Directions:

1. Preheat oven to 425 and prepare baking tray
2. Add 1 tablespoon oil to hot skillet
3. Sauté onion for 1 minute
4. Add cayenne powder, mix well into onion
5. Mix in one tablespoon apple cider vinegar and avocado pieces
6. Sauté 30-45 seconds and remove from heat
7. Lay out cabbage leaves, fill each leaf with 1 spoonful of mix
8. Lay on prepared baking tray and cook for 12-14 minutes

Nutritional Information:
Calories: 276
Total Fat: 28g
Carbohydrates: 13g
Protein: 4g

RECIPE

Ingredients:

- 10-12 asparagus spears
- 1 tablespoon of olive oil
- ½ tablespoon cayenne powder
- 1 cup plain bread crumbs
- 1 cup vegan, or parmesan cheese (optional)

Directions:

1. Preheat oven to 400 and prepare a baking tray
2. Wash and dry asparagus spears and set aside
3. In a bowl mix together the olive oil, cayenne powder, bread crumbs, and parmesan cheese
4. Using tongs or a fork roll the asparagus spears in the bowls mixture, make sure it's thoroughly covered, and lay out on the tray
5. Cook 20-23 minutes or until cheese turns golden brown

Nutrition Information:
Calories: 189
Total Fat: 8g
Carbohydrates: 9g
Protein: 5g

RECIPE

Avocado Casserole

Ingredients:
- Cubed or torn ciabatta bread
- 1 tablespoon olive oil
- 1/3 cup diced scallions
- 1/2 can diced tomatoes or fresh
- 1 large or 2 medium avocados diced
- 3 finely diced basil leaves or 1 tablespoon
- 1 teaspoon turmeric powder
- 1 cup vegan or mozzarella cheese

Directions:
1. Preheat oven to 350 and prepare a 11x9 casserole dish.
2. In a small bowl mix together olive oil, scallions, tomatoes, avocados and basil.
3. Place bread into casserole dish and top with tomato/avocado mixture.
4. Top with your choice of cheese
5. Cook uncovered 18-22 minutes.

Nutritional Information:
Calories: 387
Total Fat: 21g
Carbohydrates: 26g
Protein: 11g

Spicy Eggchilada

Ingredients:
- 2 tbsp coconut oil
- 5-7 large egg whites with yolks
- ½ can low sodium, no salt added, petite tomatoes
- 1/3 cup chunky salsa
- 1 teaspoon tobasco sauce
- 1 tablespoon cayenne powder
- 1 teaspoon cumin
- 1 teaspoon celery salt
- 1 package cheddar cheese or vegan cheese
- ½ cup fresh chopped cilantro

Directions:
1. Prepare skillet or Dutch oven over medium high heat.
2. Mix together eggs, tomatoes, salsa, hot sauce, chili powder, cumin, and celery salt. Top with cheese and let set. Periodically push a spatula under it to insure that it doesn't stick.
3. Cook, uncovered, 18-22 minutes

Nutritional Information:
Calories: 601
Total Fat: 28g
Carbohydrates: 12g
Protein: 30g

RECIPE

Marinated Eggplant

Ingredients:
- 1 tablespoon coconut oil
- 1/4 cup honey (optional)
- 1 teaspoon Worcester sauce
- 2 tblsp apple cider vinegar – w/mother
- 1 tablespoon ginger powder or minced
- 1 teaspoon black pepper
- 1 tsp turmeric
- 1 tsp sea salt
- 1 small red onion diced
- 1 – 3 diced eggplant

Directions:
1. In plastic bag mix oil, honey, ginger, pepper
2. Place eggplant and onion pieces in marinade and let sit in refrigerator 4 hours
3. Over oil sauté onions and eggplant over medium high heat 5 minutes.

Nutritional Information:
Calories: 211
Total Fat: 7g
Carbohydrates: 22g
Proteins: 2g

Avocado Brown Rice Medley

Ingredients:
- ¾ tablespoon olive oil
- 1 cup brown rice
- 1 cup water
- Garlic and parsley powder
- 1 tomato diced
- 1 white onion diced
- 1 cup eggplant diced
- 1 diced avocado
- 1/4 cup lemon juice
- 1 tablespoon diced basil

Directions:
1. Pour olive oil in a Dutch oven or large pot and let warm over high heat. Sauté tomato, onion, eggplant, and avocado for 1-2 minutes.
2. Pour lemon juice, rice, water, and garlic and parsley powder and bring to a boil stirring frequently.
3. Reduce heat to low, cover, and simmer 25 minutes stirring occasionally.

Nutritional Information:
Calories: 457
Total Fat: 18g
Carbohydrates: 34g
Protein: 6g

Notes

RECIPE

Zucchini Casserole

Ingredients:
- 2-3 zucchinis cubed in 2x2 pieces
- 1 cup vegan or mozzarella cheese
- 2 – 3 tbsp cup coconut oil
- 1/2 tablespoon parsley
- ½ tablespoon rosemary
- 1 tsp turmeric
- 1 tsp sea salt

Directions:
1. Preheat oven to 400 and prepare a 9x9 casserole dish.
2. Wash, dry, and cube zucchini; place in a bowl.
3. Pour in bowl with zucchini, cheese, oil, & spices
4. Cook 18-20 minutes.

Nutritional Information:
Calories: 377
Total Fat: 18g
Carbohydrates: 29g
Protein: 3g

Eggplant Mash

Ingredients:
- 1 lb eggplant, cut into chunks
- 3 medium golden potatoes, cut into chunks
- 1 bay leaf
- 1 tsp dried thyme
- 1 tsp smoked paprika
- 2 tbsp sweet paprika
- 2 cups vegetable broth
- 1 cup tomatoes, diced
- 1 tbsp coconut flour
- 4 garlic cloves, minced
- 1 medium white onion, diced
- 1 bell pepper, chopped
- 4 tbsp extra virgin olive oil
- Pepper
- Salt

Directions:
1. Add extra virgin olive oil into the large pot and heat over medium heat.
2. Add eggplant to the pot and sauté for 10 minutes or until lightly browned.
3. Add garlic, onion, and bell pepper into the pot and sauté for 5 minutes.
4. Sprinkle flour over vegetables and stir until vegetables are well coated.
5. Add potatoes, bay leaf, thyme, smoked paprika, sweet paprika, broth, and tomatoes to the pot and stir well.
6. Turn heat to high and bring to simmer.

7. Reduce heat to low and remove the cover and simmer for 20 minutes or until potatoes are tender.
8. Remove pot from heat and season with pepper and salt.
9. Discard bay leaf and serve.

Nutritional Information:
Calories 332
Fat 15 g
Carbohydrates 44 g
Protein 8 g

RECIPE

Bok Choy Jasmin Rice Medley

Ingredients:
- 1 cup jasmine rice
- 1 tablespoon apple cider vinegar
- 1/3 cup organic honey
- ½ teaspoon black pepper
- ½ teaspoon cayenne powder
- 1 finely diced bok choy
- 1 cup fajita peppers and onions

Directions:
1. Preheat oven to 350 and prepare 9x9 casserole dish.
2. Put one cup of rice in bottom of dish; pour in apple cider vinegar and honey.
3. Wash, dry, and dice on stalk of bok choy.
4. Place bok choy, fajitas, onions, black pepper, and cayenne powder on top of rice.
5. Cover with foil and cook for 30 minutes.

Nutritional Information:
Calories: 201
Total Fat: 2g
Carbohydrates: 30g
Proteins: 5 g

Spring Rolls

Ingredients:
* 6-7 rice paper wrappers
* 1/2 cup carrot matchsticks
* 1/2 cup sliced cucumber
* 1 cup diced avocado
* 1 teaspoon white wine vinegar
* 1 teaspoon lemon juice
* ½ tablespoon apple cider vinegar
* 1 tsp sea salt

Directions:
1. Preheat oven to 350 and prepare baking tray.
2. Layout wrappers on tray.
3. In a bowl mix together carrots, cucumber, avocado, vinegar, lemon juice, salt, and apple cider vinegar
4. Place 1 spoonful of mixture into each wrapper and roll up
5. Cook 30 minutes

Nutritional Information:
Calories: 323
Total Fat: 16
Carbohydrates: 9 g
Protein: 6 g

Notes

RECIPE

Ingredients:
- 1 lb eggplant, 1/4 inch thick slices
- 1 lb button mushrooms, clean and sliced
- 1/2 tsp red pepper flakes
- 1/2 tsp dried oregano
- 1 tbsp fresh rosemary
- 2 tbsp capers
- 1/2 cup tomatoes, crushed
- 14 oz can tomatoes, diced
- 1/2 cup vegetable stock
- 3 garlic cloves, minced
- 1 bell pepper, sliced
- 1 small white onion, sliced
- 6 oz dried penne pasta
- 3 tbsp olive oil
- Pepper
- Salt

Directions:
1. Preheat the oven to 400 F.
2. Line baking tray with parchment paper.
3. Rub 1 tbsp olive oil on eggplant slices and place slices on baking tray.
4. Bake eggplant in preheated oven for 20 minutes. Remove from oven and set aside to cool.
5. Cook pasta according to the packet instruction. Drain pasta well and set aside.
6. Add 1 tbsp olive oil into the pan and heat over medium heat.

7. Add mushroom in the pan and sauté for 5 minutes on each side. Transfer mushroom to a plate and set aside.
8. Add remaining olive oil to the pan.
9. Add bell pepper and onion and sauté for 5 minutes.
10. Add garlic and sauté for 1 minute.
11. Add stock and bring to simmer. Allow cooking until liquid is half.
12. Add red pepper flakes, oregano, rosemary, capers, tomatoes, and diced tomatoes to the pan and stir well and cook for 5 minutes.
13. Stir baked eggplant into the mixture and cook for 5 minutes.
14. Remove pan from heat and season with pepper and salt.
15. Divide cooked pasta into 4 serving dishes and top with eggplant mixture.
16. Serve and enjoy.

Nutritional Information:
Calories 317
Fat 12 g
Carbohydrates 45 g
Protein 3g

Notes

RECIPE

Ingredients:
- 2/3 cup low sodium chickpeas
- 1/2 tablespoon olive oil or coconut oil
- 1 teaspoon red pepper flakes
- 1 teaspoon chopped oregano
- 1/2 teaspoon thyme

Directions:
1. Rinse chickpeas and drain
2. Put all chickpeas, oil, red pepper flakes, oregano, and thyme in food processor and blend.
3. Store in an airtight container in the refrigerator; will keep 3-5 days.
4. Serve as a topping, or dip.

Nutritional Information:
Calories: 145
Total Fat 7.5:
Carbohydrates: 35.3 mg
Protein: 8.3 g

Notes

RECIPE

Stuffed Peppers

Ingredients:
- 1 cup cauliflower mash (instructions below)
- ¾ tablespoon melted butter, or coconut oil
- 1/3 tablespoon minced garlic or garlic powder
- 4 bell peppers – any color
- 1/2 cup eggplant cubed, diced
- 1 teaspoon basil
- ½ teaspoon oregano

Directions:
1. Preheat oven to 350 and prepare 9x9 casserole dish
2. Wash, dry, and remove the ribs and seeds from the peppers. Put in dish when done.
3. In a food processor add cauliflower, oil or butter, and garlic and puree until a mashed potato consistency is achieved
4. Spoon mixture in peppers
5. Top with pieces of eggplant, basil, oregano, and cheese
6. Bake, covered, 25-30 minutes.

Nutritional Information:
Calories: 174
Total Fat: 10g
Carbohydrates: 7g
Protein: 3

Chickpea Casserole

Ingredients:
- 1 can low sodium chickpeas
- 1 teaspoon olive oil
- 1 cup water
- 1/4 cup dry white wine or cooking white wine
- 2 teaspoon chili powder
- 1 teaspoon red pepper flakes
- 1 cup uncooked brown rice

Directions:
1. Drain beans and wash
2. Put all ingredients in crockpot
3. Cook on high 1 hour
4. Or, cook rice on stove with 2 cups water. Boil for 15 minutes, then drain.
5. Heat oil in pan. Add all ingredients accept rice.
6. Cook medium heat 10 minutes, then add rice.
7. Cook and stir until mixed well.

Nutritional Information:
Calories: 223
Total Fat: 5g
Carbohydrates: 24g
Protein: 5g

Notes

Tofu Fajitas

Ingredients:
- 4 corn tortilla shells, warmed
- 1 tablespoon coconut oil
- 1 large sweet onion, cut into strips and caramelized
- 2 bell peppers sliced into strips
- 14 oz firm tofu
- 2 teaspoon lemon juice
- 1 teaspoon cayenne pepper
- ½ teaspoon cumin

Directions:
1. Paint some oil on each side of the corn shell, warm shell in skillet 2-3 minutes on each side. Can keep warm if wrapped in aluminum foil and kept in 200 degree oven.
2. Wash, dry, and cut into strips onions, peppers, and tofu.
3. In large pot let oil mix over med. High heat.
4. Add onion strip and sauté stirring until a brown-gold and very fragrant, approx. 2-3 minutes. Add peppers and tofu and cook approx. 1 minute. Remove and drain

Nutritional Information:
Calories: 511
Total Fat: 26g
Carbohydrates: 29g
Protein: 33g

RECIPE

Variation ideas – Schedules - Notes

Tofu Basil Eggplant

Ingredients:
- 1 large Italian eggplant, cut into 3/4 inch slices
- 4 tbsp coconut oil
- 2 garlic cloves, minced
- 14 oz firm tofu, block
- 1 red onion, sliced
- 1 green bell pepper, sliced
- 1 red bell pepper, sliced
- 1 yellow bell pepper, sliced
- Basil leaves
- For sauce:
- 2 tsp cornstarch
- 2 tsp chili sauce
- 1/4 cup water
- 1/2 cup tamari
- 4.5 tbsp Hoisin sauce

Directions:
1. Cut eggplant slices into 2 to 3 pieces each.
2. Heat 2 tbsp coconut oil in a pan over medium heat.
3. Add eggplant pieces into the pan and coat well with oil.
4. Add little water to the pan and cover and cook eggplant.
5. Stir eggplant pieces every few minutes.
6. Once the eggplant is cooked then turn off the heat and set pan aside.
7. Cut tofu into the pieces and squeeze out excess liquid from tofu.
8. Heat 1 tbsp oil in a pan over medium heat.
9. Add tofu to the pan and cook until golden brown.
10. Transfer cooked tofu to the eggplant pan.

11. Heat remaining oil in a pan and sauté bell peppers and onion and crispy. Add garlic and sauté for a minute.
12. Transfer onion and bell pepper mixture to the eggplant and tofu pan.
13. Whisk all sauce ingredients together.
14. Heat eggplant mixture pan over medium heat.
15. Once the pan is hot then add sauce mixture over veggies and mix well and cook for few minutes.
16. Remove pan from heat and add chopped basil.
17. Stir well and serve.

Nutritional Information:
Calories 504
Fat 32 g
Carbohydrates 26 g
Protein 19 g

RECIPE

Veggie Pita Pockets

Ingredients:
- 1 small, low sodium, pita pocket halved
- 1 teaspoon smoky paprika
- 1/4 teaspoon black pepper
- 1/3 cup diced bok choy pieces
- 1 diced avocado pieces
- 1/3 cup diced cucumber pieces
- 1/3 cup matchstick carrots
- 1/3 cup diced cherry tomatoes
- 1 teaspoon lemon juice

Directions:
1. Turn on broiler onto high and prepare baking tray
2. Wash, dry, and dice all vegetables.
3. Put vegetables into a bowl, add spices, and lemon juice; mix well.
4. Spoon mix inside pita's and warm in broiler 2-4 minutes.

Nutritional Information:
Calories: 512
Total Fat: 23g
Carbohydrates: 56g
Protein: 12g

Notes

RECIPE

Gout Friendly Pizza

Ingredients:
- 2 tablespoon olive oil
- 1 cup Feta cheese crumbled (vegan cheese is optional)
- 4 cup cherry tomatoes, halved and halved again
- 1 cup radish, diced
- 1 avocado, diced
- 1/3 cup diced low sodium black olives (optional)
- 1 teaspoon red pepper flakes
- 1 tablespoon coarsely chopped basil leaves
- 1 teaspoon oregano
- 1 low sodium or no sodium small pizza shell, pizza dough, or flatbread (flatbread my favorite)

Directions:
1. Lay out dough and using a sauce brush 'paint' with olive oil
2. Sprinkle with seasoning and cheese
3. Add remaining ingredients.
4. Bake according to shell/dough instructions.

Nutritional Information:
Calories: 524
Total Fat: 19g
Carbohydrates: 45 g
Protein: 13 g

RECIPE

Baked Tofu and Roasted Peppers

Ingredients:
- 1 tbsp Olive oil
- 1/2 shallot diced
- 7 to 14 oz firm tofu, cubed and dried
- 1/3 cup water
- 1 tablespoon dry white wine or white cooking wine
- 1 teaspoon red pepper slices
- 1 tsp turmeric

Directions:
1. Preheat oven to 400 and prepare a 9x9 casserole dish
2. Wash, dry, and prepare shallots, tofu, and peppers for baking
3. Place ingredients into dish
4. Cook 20-25 minutes.

Nutritional Information:
Calories: 456
Total Fat: 27 g
Carbohydrates: 24 g
Protein: 8 g

Notes

RECIPE

Eggplant Chickpea

Ingredients:

- 1 large eggplant, cut into pieces
- 15 oz can chickpeas, drained and rinsed
- 1/4 tsp cayenne pepper
- 1/4 tsp smoked paprika
- 1/4 tsp turmeric
- 1/2 tsp ground cumin
- 1 tsp onion powder
- 1 tbsp curry powder
- 1 cup coconut milk
- 2 garlic cloves, minced
- 1/2 red onion, diced
- Pepper
- Salt

Directions:

1. Add onion and eggplant into the large pan and cook over medium heat for 5 minutes. Add garlic and for a minute.
2. Add chickpea to the pan and stir well.
3. Add coconut milk, spices, pepper, and salt. Stir well and simmer for 5 minutes.
4. Stir well and serve.

Nutritional Information:
Calories 521
Fat 6 g
Carbohydrates 75 g
Protein 16 g

Notes

RECIPE

Kale and Tofu

Ingredients:

- 6 fresh kale leaves
- 6oz. firm tofu cubes
- Olive oil for drizzling
- No-salt seasoning (Mrs Dash is great)

Directions:

1. Prepare baking tray and preheat oven to 400.
2. Layout individual kale leaves, drop one tofu cube in the center. Fold leaf ends over tofu cube and flip.
3. Drizzle with olive oil and seasoning
4. Bake 18-22 minutes.

Nutritional Information:
Calories: 337
Total Fat: 12
Carbohydrates: 16
Protein: 9 g

RECIPE

Stuffed Pepper Melts

Ingredients:
- 1 tablespoon of coconut oil
- 4 bell peppers, cleaned and hollowed
- 1 cup cauliflower rice
- 1 caramelized scallion
- 3 tablespoons diced mushrooms(baby portabello)
- 1 diced habanero or jalapeno pepper
- 1 cup feta crumbled or Vegan cheese

Directions:
1. Prepare a 9x9 baking dish and preheat the oven to 325
2. In a large mixing bowl mix together all ingredients, except the cheese, and spoon into hollowed out peppers.
3. Top with cheese, place in dish and cook, uncovered, 20-25 minutes.

Nutritional Information:
Calories: 207
Total Fat: 12 g
Carbohydrates: 16g
Protein: 2 g

Notes

RECIPE

Marinated Mint Eggplant

Ingredients:
- 2 large eggplant, cut into 1/4 inch slices
- 1 tbsp rice vinegar
- 4 tbsp olive oil
- 2 – 4 garlic cloves, chopped
- 1/4 cup fresh mint, chopped
- 1 tbsp oregano
- 1 teaspoon cayenne pepper
- Salt to taste

Directions:
1. Add sliced eggplant into the mixing bowl.
2. Sprinkle a little salt over the slices eggplant and set aside for 30 minutes to release some water.
3. Rinse eggplant well and pat dry with paper towel.
4. Brush eggplant with oil.
5. Place eggplant slices on the hot griddle pan and cook until softened.
6. In a small bowl, mix together all remaining ingredients and set aside.
7. Arrange cooked eggplant slices on serving dish and drizzle marinade over the eggplant slices.
8. Serve and enjoy.

Nutritional Information:
Calories 234
Fat 18 g
Carbohydrates 10 g
Protein 1 g

RECIPE

Spiced Eggplant

Ingredients:
- 3 medium eggplants, sliced into wedges
- 1/2 cup basil, chopped
- 4 green onions, chopped
- 2 bell pepper, cut into strips
- 8 oz button mushrooms, sliced
- 2 tbsp coconut oil
- 1 tbsp salt
- For sauce:
- 1/4 cup vegetable broth
- 1 tbsp rice vinegar
- 1 tbsp soy sauce
- 2 tbsp tamari
- 1/4 cup brown sugar (optional)
- 1/4 cup sweet chili sauce
- 2 tbsp chili paste
- 3 garlic cloves, minced

Directions:
1. Add eggplant into the bowl and sprinkle salt over the eggplant and set aside for 15 minutes.
2. Rinse eggplant slices and pat dry with paper towel.
3. In a bowl, whisk all sauce ingredients together.
4. heat coconut oil in the pan over medium-high heat.
5. Add eggplant and cook until it is tender.
6. Remove eggplant from pan and place on a plate.
7. Add green onion, mushrooms, and bell peppers into the pan and sauté for 5 minutes.
8. Add eggplant and sauce. Let simmer for 10 minutes.
9. Add basil and stir well.

10. Serve and enjoy.

Nutritional Value (Amount per Serving):
Calories 333
Fat 12 g
Carbohydrates 21 g
Protein 2 g

Notes

RECIPE

Eggplant with Quinoa

Ingredients:
- 1 large eggplant, cut into 1-inch cubes
- 1 1/2 cups cooked quinoa
- 5 oz fresh baby spinach
- 2 garlic cloves, chopped
- 3 tbsp olive oil
- Pepper
- Salt

Directions:
1. Preheat the oven to 420 F.
2. Spray a baking tray with cooking spray and set aside.
3. In a mixing bowl, add eggplant with 2 tbsp olive oil. Season eggplant with pepper and salt.
4. Spread eggplant onto baking tray and roast in preheated oven for 20-25 minutes.
5. Heat remaining oil in a pan over medium heat.
6. Add garlic and spinach to the pan and cook until spinach is wilted. Remove pan from heat.
7. Once the eggplant is roast then remove from oven and add in spinach pan.
8. Add cooked quinoa to the pan and mix well.
9. Serve and enjoy.

Nutritional Information:
Calories 364
Fat 14 g
Carbohydrates 29 g
Protein 11 g

Notes

Red Potato Mix

Ingredients:

- 2 red potatoes (peeled and cubed)
- 1 carrot (chopped)
- 1 red onion (finely chopped)
- ½ cup frozen green beans (thawed)
- 10 French style green beans (cubed)
- 2 tomatoes (blanched, peeled and chopped)
- 1 tsp mustard seed
- 1 tsp ground cumin
- ½ tsp garlic powder
- ½ tsp ground ginger
- ½ tsp ground turmeric
- ½ tsp chili powder
- 1 tsp garam masala
- 1 sprig cilantro leaves (for garnishing)
- 1 quart water (cold)
- 1 tsp sea salt
- 1 tbsp olive oil

Directions:

1. In a large bowl, soak the carrots, green beans and potatoes in cold water for an hour. Drain.
2. Place the carrots, green beans, peas, potatoes, salt and turmeric in a microwave safe dish and cook for approximately 8 minutes.
3. In a large skillet, heat the oil over medium heat. Cook mustard seeds and cumin; when seeds start to sputter and pop add the onion and sauté until transparent.
4. Stir in the tomatoes, garam masala, ginger, garlic and chili powder and sauté for about 2-3 minutes.

5. Add the cooked vegetables to the tomato mixture and sauté for an additional minute or two.
6. Garnish with cilantro leaves and serve.

Nutritional Information:
Calories 350
Fat 8 g
Carbohydrates 43
Protein 3 g

RECIPE

Potato Spinach Casserole

Ingredients:
- 5 russet potatoes (peeled and quatered)
- 1 cup baby spinach (chopped)
- 1 celery stalk (chopped)
- 1 bunch of parsley (chopped)
- 1 green onion (chopped)
- 1 red onion (diced)
- 1 garlic clove (crushed)
- 1 tbsp tamari
- 1 bay leaf
- 8 whole black peppercorns
- 1 cup corn kernels
- 1 tsp paprika
- ½ pound shitake mushrooms (sliced)
- 1 pound firm tofu (crumbled)
- 1 tbsp light miso paste
- 4 tbsp olive oil (extra virgin)
- 1 cube vegetable bouillon
- 1/8 cup coconut flour

Directions:
1. Preheat the oven to 400 degrees F.
2. Fill a large pot with water and place the peeled potatoes inside it. Add in the celery, parsley, garlic, peppercorn, onion and the bay leaf.
3. Bring the mixture to boil and then simmer over medium low heat for 15 to 20 minutes or until the potatoes become tender.

4. In a large skillet, heat about 1 tablespoon of olive oil and sauté the onion and garlic in it over medium heat. Add in the mushrooms and sauté for another 2 to 3 minutes.
5. Crumble the tofu into chunks and add into the skillet to the filling mixture. Mix well.
6. Stir in the paprika, and tamari. Mix well and sauté the filling mixture while stirring frequently for approximately 20 minutes over medium heat.
7. Transfer potatoes from water to a large bowl, reserving 3 1/2 cups of the remaining stock. Add miso, oil, and 3/4 to 1 cup of the potato stock to the potatoes a little at a time, mashing potatoes as you add the stock. Adding only enough water to moisten potatoes.
8. Add the corn and the spinach to the filling mixture and mix well.
9. Spoon the filling into an oiled casserole dish and pat it down with the back of a large spoon.
10. Spread the potato crust evenly over the filling and smooth out the top with a spatula.
11. Sprinkle the paprika on top and bake in the oven for 30 to 40 minutes or until the crust turns golden.
12. While the casserole bakes prepare the gravy by heating a spoon ful of olive oil in a frying pan. Add the flour and yeast and stir over medium heat until it forms a paste.
13. Stir in the reserved 2 ½ cups of potato water and mix until the gravy thickens.
14. Add the instant gravy mix and continue to whisk.
15. Serve the casserole with crust on the bottom and the filling on top followed by a scoop of gravy.

Nutritional Information:
Calories: 739
Fat: 18
Carbohydrates: 89
Protein: 24

Notes

RECIPE

Mushroom Kabobs

Ingredients:
- ¾ cup fresh button mushrooms (sliced)
- 1 green bell pepper (cut into 1 inch pieces)
- 2 red bell peppers (chopped)
- 1 garlic clove (minced)
- 2 tsp thyme (chopped)
- 1 tsp rosemary (chopped)
- 2 tbsp lemon juice
- 4 tblsp olive oil
- 1/4 tsp sea salt
- 1/4 teaspoon ground black pepper

Directions:
1. Preheat the grill at medium heat.
2. Thread the mushrooms and peppers on to the skewers.
3. In a mixing bowl, whisk together olive oil with garlic, rosemary, salt, pepper, thyme and lemon juice.
4. Brush the mushrooms and peppers with olive oil.
5. Place the kabobs on the grill and cook for approximately 4 to 6 minutes or until the mushrooms are cooked.

Nutritional Information:
Calories: 143
Fat: 18
Carbohydrates: 12 g
Protein: 2

Notes

RECIPE

Garbanzo Curry

Ingredients:

- ¾ tsp. extra-virgin olive oil
- ¼ red onion, minced
- ½ clove garlic, minced
- ¼ tsp. fresh ginger root, finely chopped
- 1 whole clove
- 1/4 tsp. cinnamon
- 1/8 tsp. ground cumin
- 1/8 tsp ground coriander.
- Pinch of salt
- 1 tsp. cayenne pepper
- 1 tsp. ground turmeric
- 15oz-can garbanzo beans, drained and rinsed.
- 2 Tbsp. chopped fresh cilantro
- 1/4 cup jasmine rice
- 1/2 cup water

Directions:

1.	First prepare the rice by placing both the rice and water in a medium saucepan or small pot. Turn the heat to high until it begins to boil, and then reduce to low, cover and let simmer for 15 minutes.

2.	Heat olive oil in a large frying pan over medium heat for 1 minute. Sauté onions until tender, about 3-4 minutes.

3.	Stir in garlic, ginger, clove, cinnamon, cumin, coriander, salt, cayenne, and turmeric. Cook for 1 minute over medium heat, stirring constantly.

4.	Add in garbanzo beans and a little bit of water (about ½ Tbsp.).

5.	Continue to cook for, stirring occasionally, for about 15-20 minutes, or until all the ingredients are well-blended and cooked through. Remove from heat.
6.	Place cooked rice in a bowl, top with garbanzo curry, and garnish with cilantro.

Nutritional Information
Calories: 294.9
Total Fat: 4g
Carbohydrates: 56g
Protein: 7g

Ginger Stir-Fry with Coconut Rice

Ingredients:

- 1/2 clove garlic, crushed
- 1/2 tsp. chopped fresh ginger root, divided
- 2 tsp. extra virgin olive-oil, divided
- 1/4 cup broccoli florets
- 1 Tbsp. snow peas
- 2 Tbsp. julienned carrots
- 1 Tbsp. red bell pepper, diced
- 1 tsp. soy sauce
- 1 tsp. water
- 1/2 chopped white onion
- 1/4 cup jasmine rice
- 1/4 cup coconut milk
- 1/4 cup water
- Sriracha (or other hot sauce)

Directions:

1. First prepare the rice by placing the rice, coconut milk, and water in a medium saucepan or small pot. Turn the heat to high until it begins to boil, and then reduce to low, cover and let simmer for 15 minutes, or until most of the coconut milk has been absorbed.

2. In a large bowl, blend garlic, half the ginger, and 1 tsp. olive oil.

3. Add the broccoli, snow peas, carrots, and bell pepper, tossing to lighting coat.

4. Heat the remaining olive oil in a wok over medium heat. Add vegetables, cook for 1 minute, stirring constantly to prevent burning.

5.	Add onions, salt, remaining ginger, soy sauce and water. Cook until vegetables are tender, but still crisp—about 2 minutes.

6.	Place coconut rice in a bowl, top with ginger stir fry. Add Sriracha to taste.

Nutritional Information
Calories: 338
Total Fat: 16 g
Carbohydrates: 42 g
Protein: 6g

RECIPE

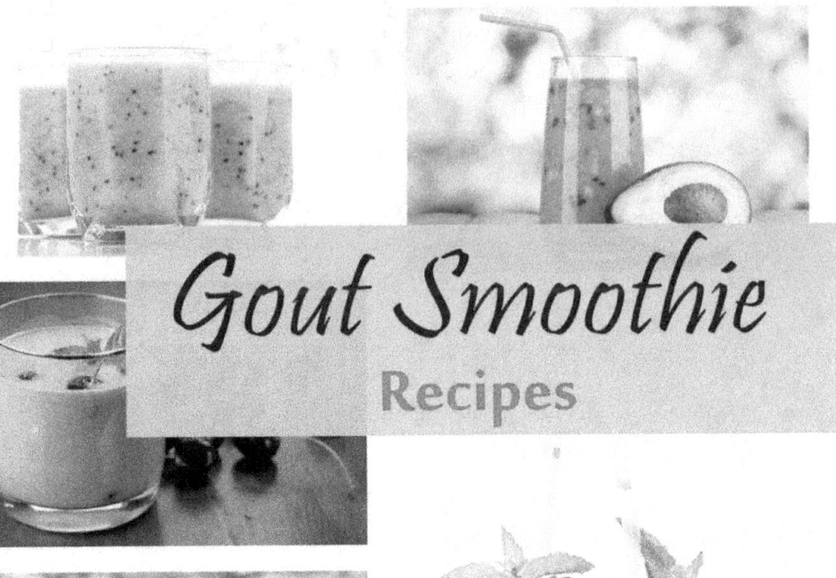

Gout Smoothie
Recipes

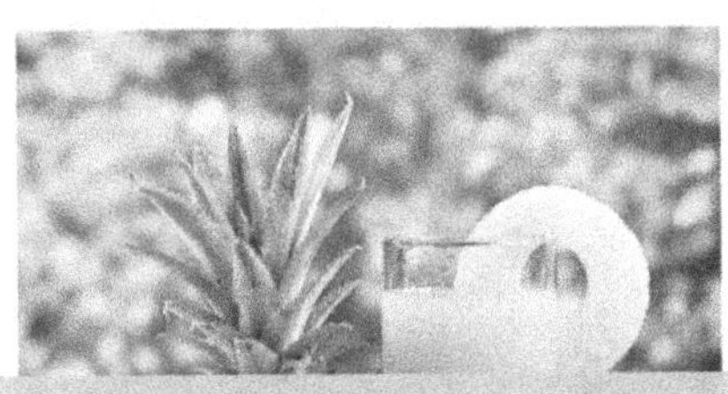

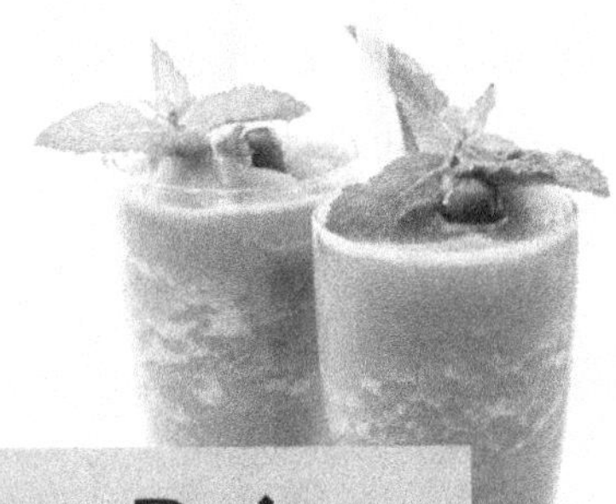

Plant Based & Non Dairy
Healthy & Anti - Inflammatory
Peter Voit

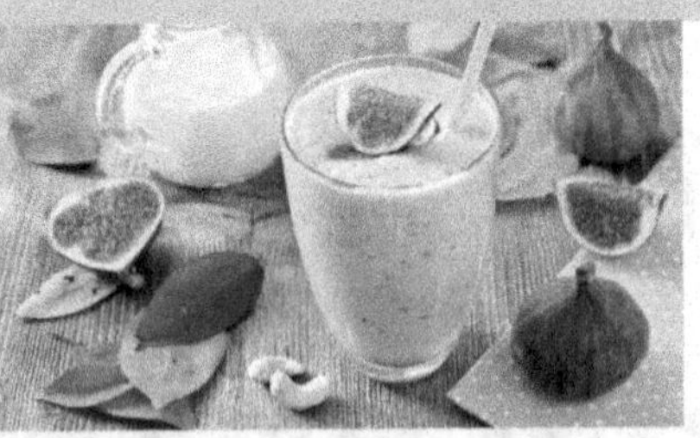

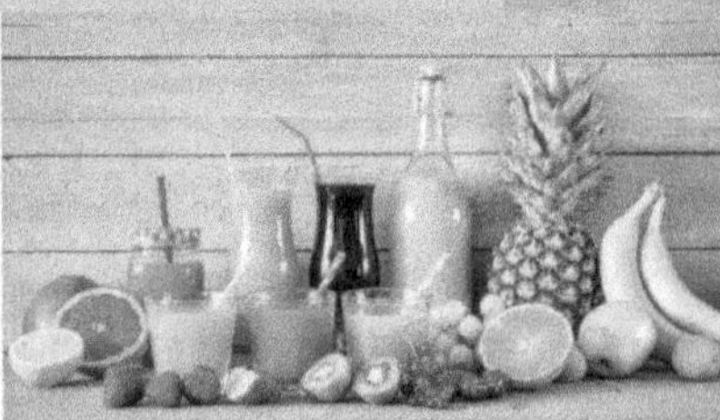

Lime – Strawberry – Spinach Smoothie

Ingredients:

- 1 lime juice
- 2 – 3 cups baby spinach
- 1 tbsp hemp seeds
- 1 cup coconut water
- 1/2 cup strawberries
- 1 banana

Directions:

1. Add lime juice, spinach, coconut water, strawberries and banana into the blender, with ice if desired, and blend until smooth.
2. Pour into the glasses and top with hemp seed.
3. Serve immediately and enjoy.

Nutritional Value (Amount per Serving):

- Calories 200

- Fat 3 g

- Carbohydrates 40 g

- Protein 3 g

Baby spinach is one of my go to greens! I just love using it inside smoothies. It is a great way to get in more vegetables!

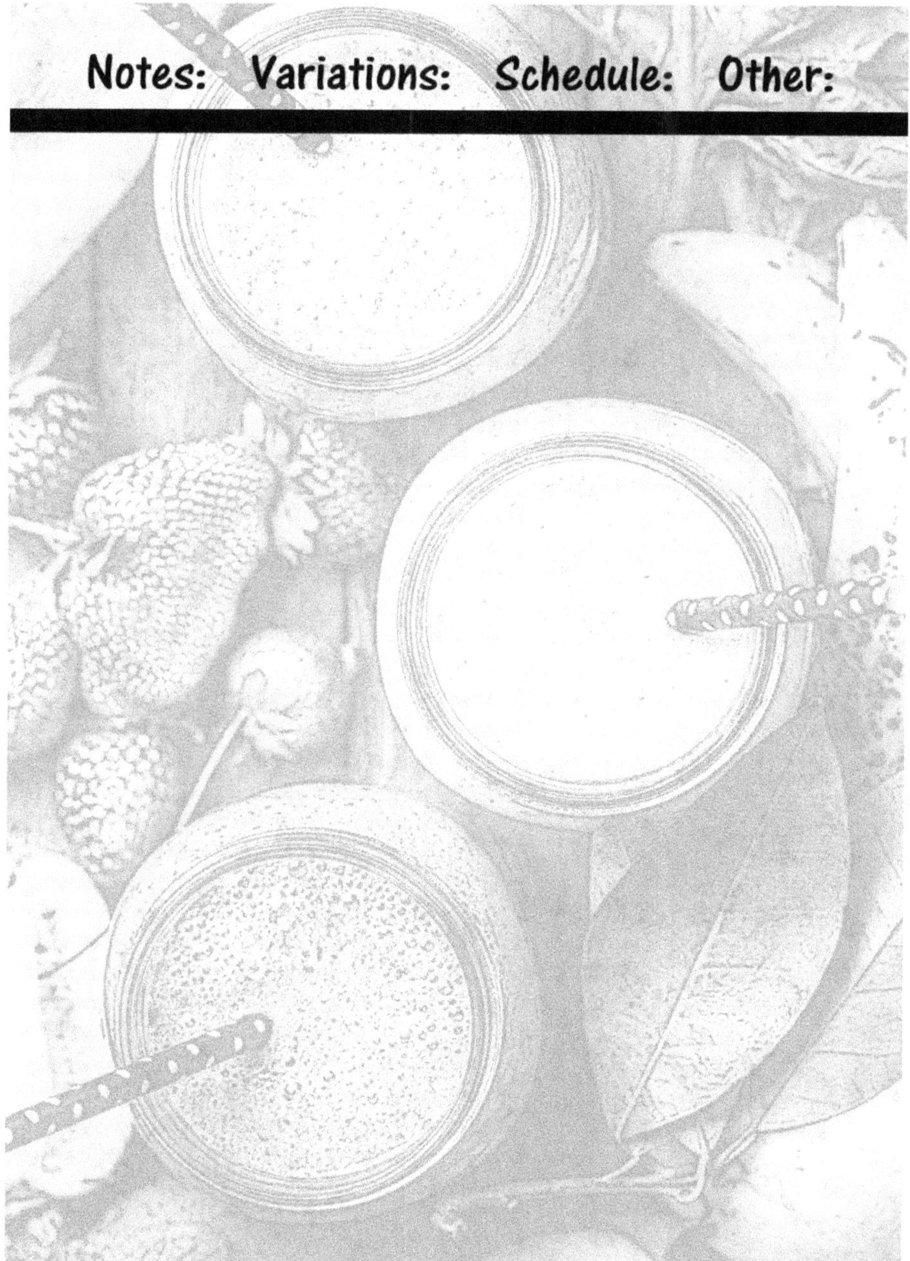

Lime – Honeydew Smoothie

Ingredients:

- 1 squeezed lime
- 2 1/2 cups honeydew
- 1 cup coconut water

Directions:

1. Add all ingredients into the blender, with ice, and blend until smooth.

Nutritional Value (Amount per Serving):

- Calories 187
- Fat 1 g
- Carbohydrates 40 g
- Protein 1 g

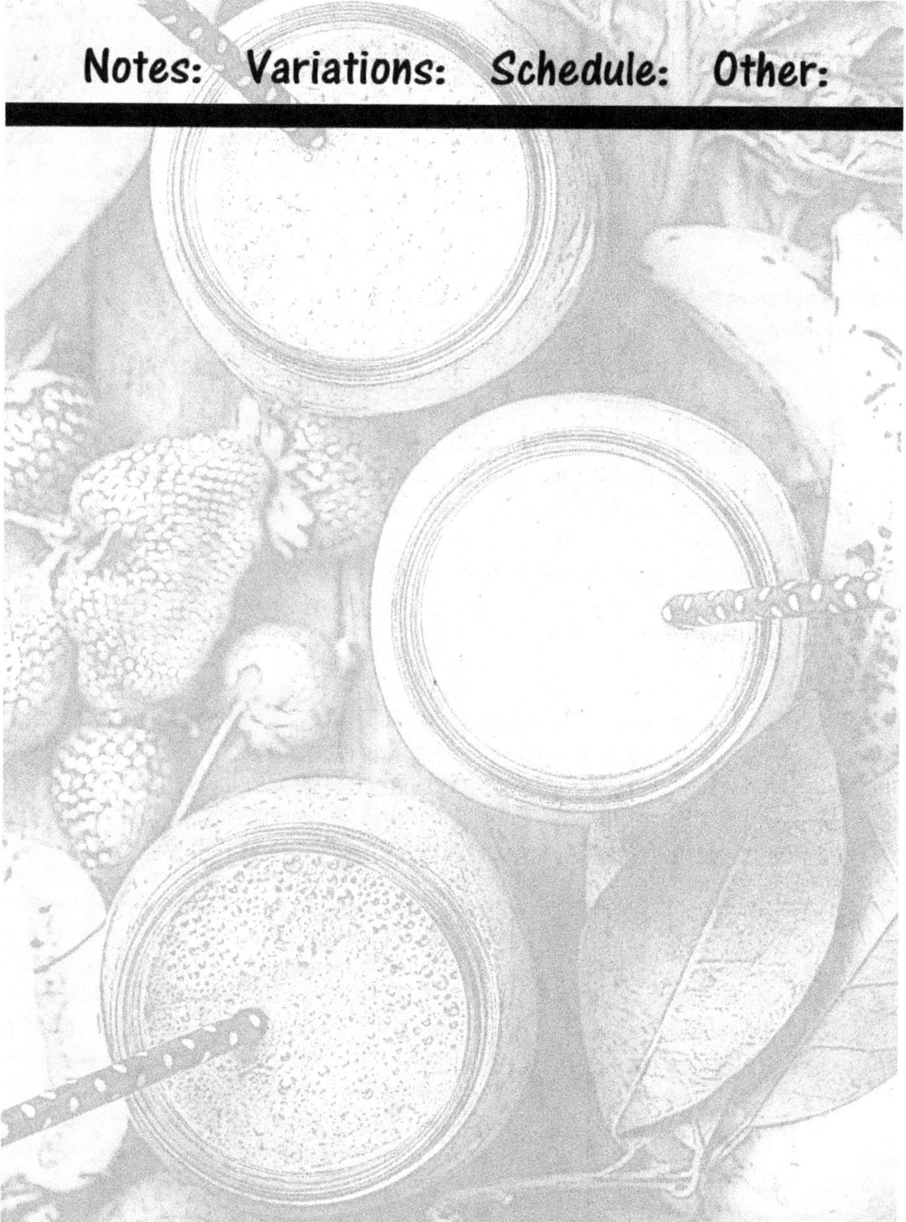

Orange – Peach – Raspberry Smoothie

Ingredients:

- 1 cups fresh orange juice(squeezed if possible)
- 2 peaches, peeled and sliced
- 1 cups almond milk
- 1 cup raspberries

Directions:

1. Add all ingredients, with desired ice into the blender and blend until smooth.

Nutritional Value (Amount per Serving):

- Calories 385
- Fat 4 g
- Carbohydrates 80 g
- Protein 4 g

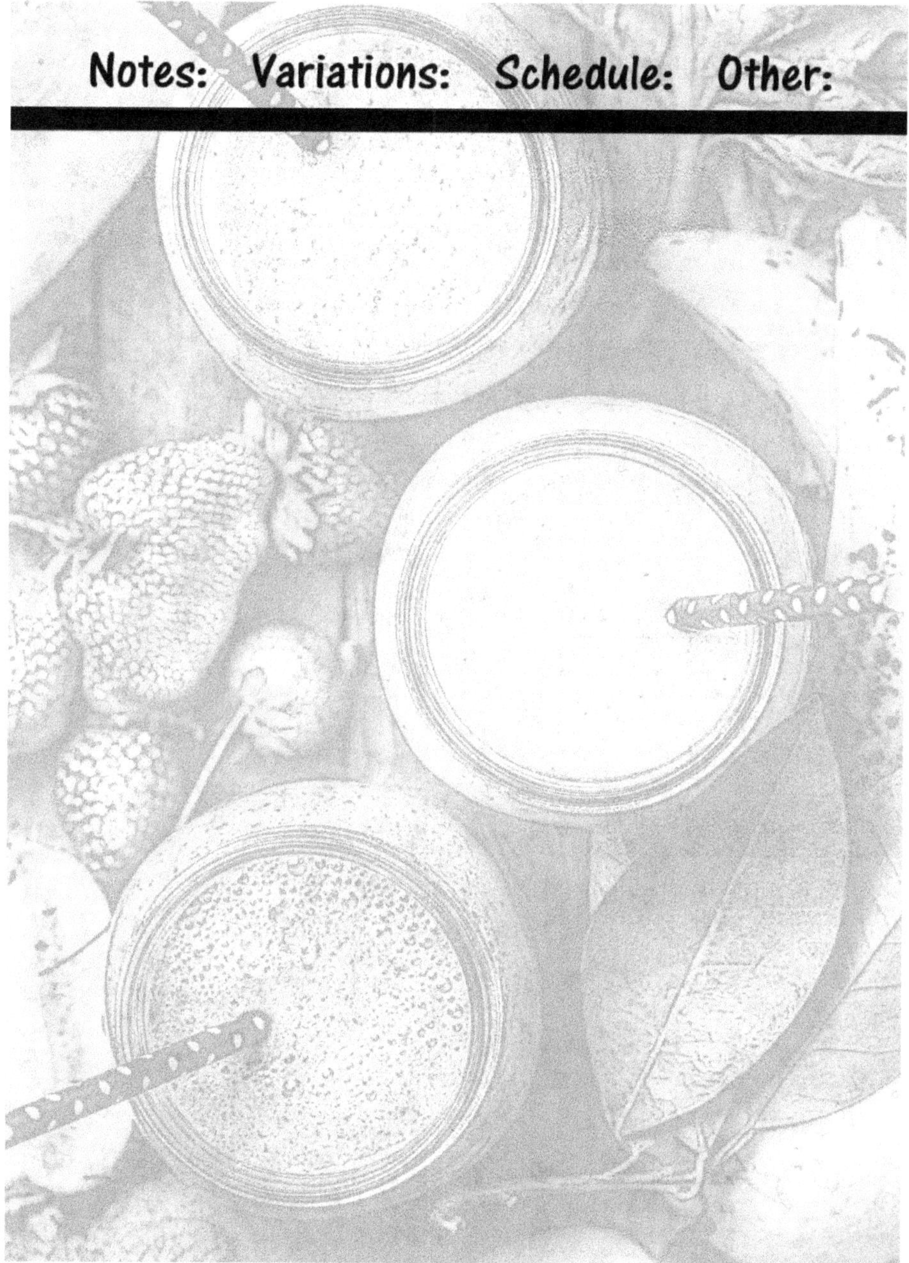

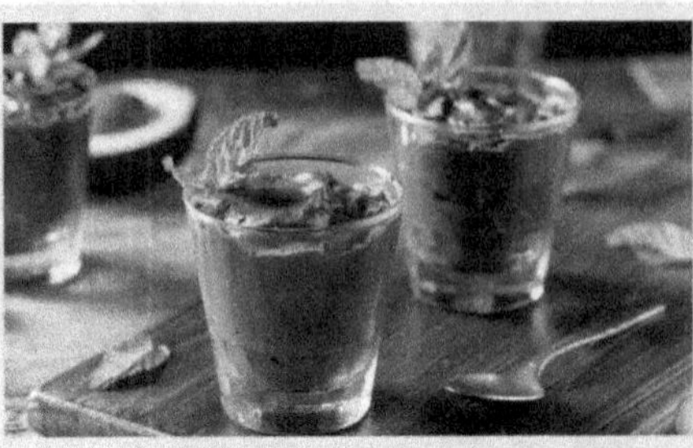

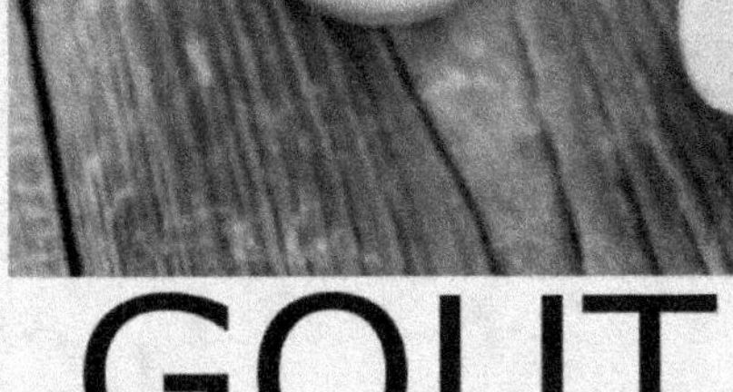

Anti - Inflammatory
Spice Turmeric In Every
Smoothie!

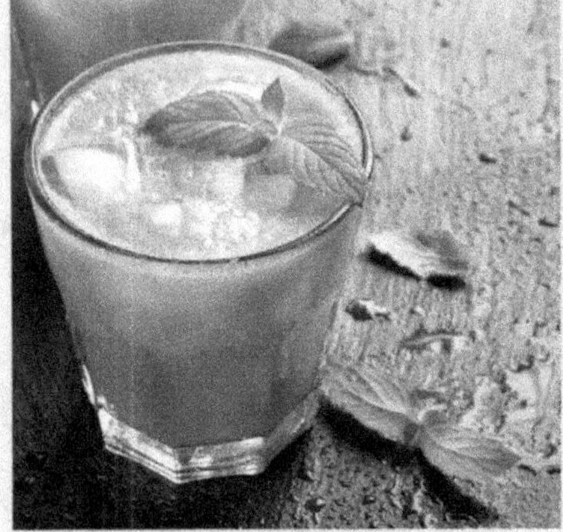

GOUT
Smoothie Recipes
Peter Voit

Delicious, & Healthy Plant
Based Smoothies!

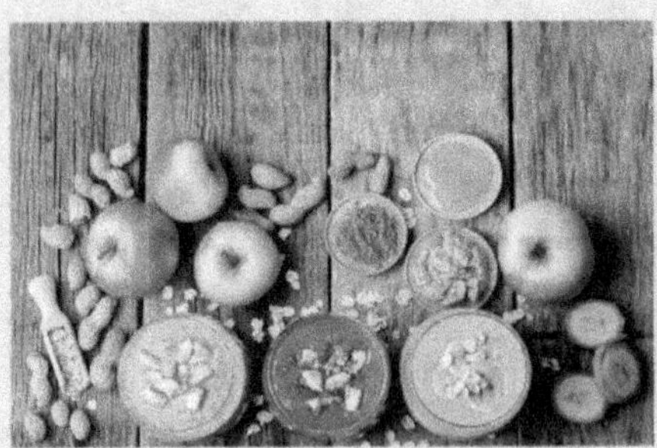

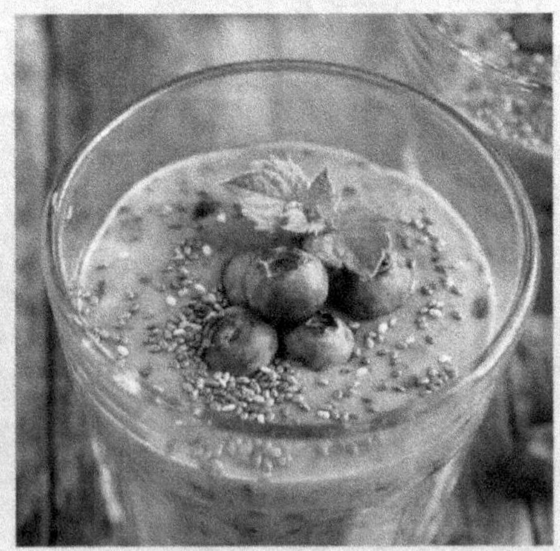

Vanilla - Cinnamon Smoothie

Ingredients

- 2 oranges, peeled and separated
- 1 cup cantaloupe chunks, peeled
- 1 cup vanilla almond milk, unsweetened
- ½ tsp. freshly grated ginger
- ½ tsp. cinnamon
- 1 – 2 tsp turmeric powder
- 4-6 ice cubes

Directions

1. Combine ingredients in a blender. Cover and blend until smooth.
2. Serve & enjoy!

Nutritional Information (per serving)

- Calories 223
- Fat 2 g
- Carbohydrates 50 g
- Protein 2 g

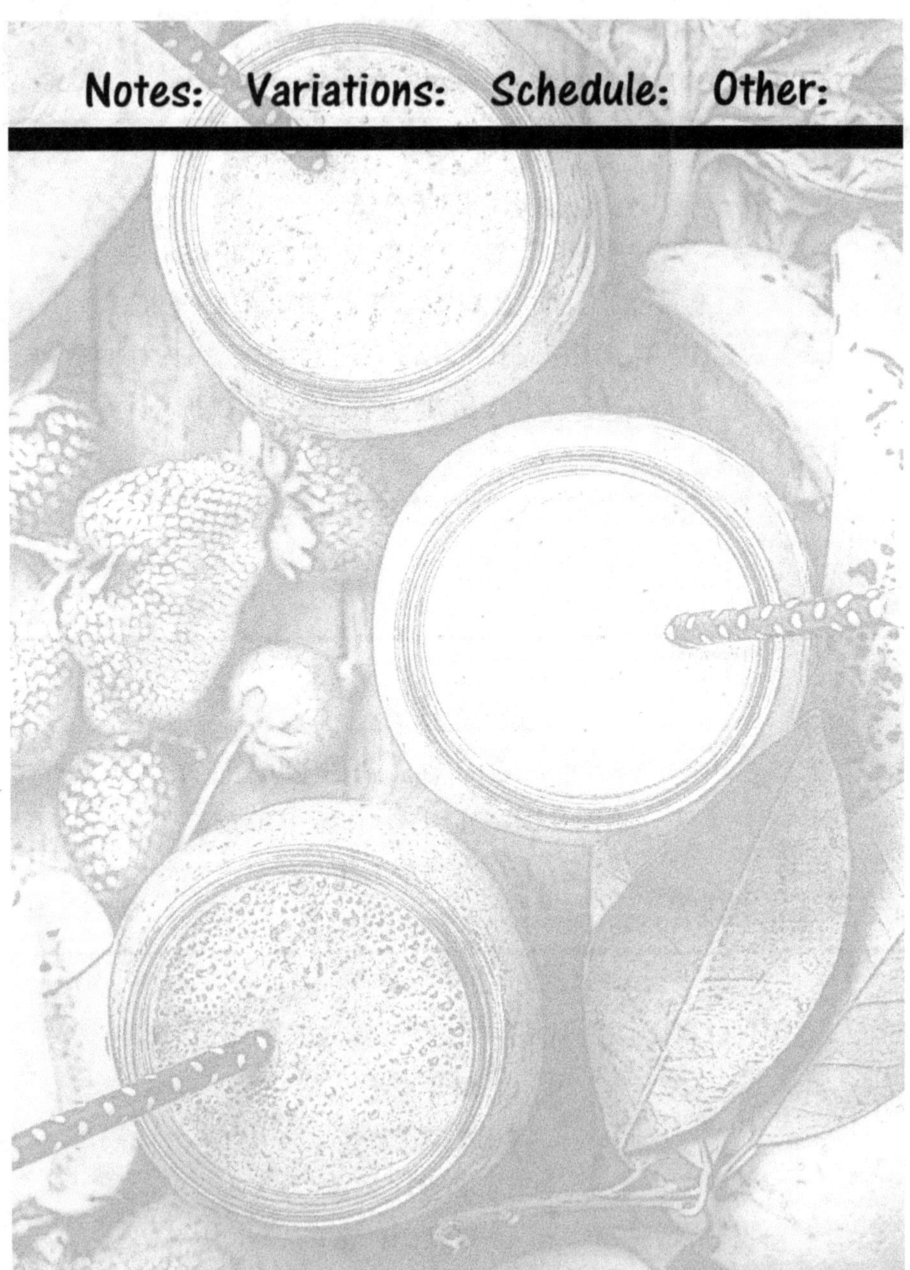

Minty Pineapple Smoothie

Ingredients
- 1 cup frozen pineapple, unsweetened
- 1 small banana, peeled
- ½ cup coconut water
- 1 lime peeled
- 3 mint leaves
- 1 – 2 tsp turmeric powder
- 4 ice cubes

Directions
1. Combine ingredients in a blender. Cover and blend until smooth.
2. Serve & enjoy!

Nutritional Information (per serving)
- Calories 210
- Fat 1 g
- Carbohydrates 49 g
- Protein 1 g

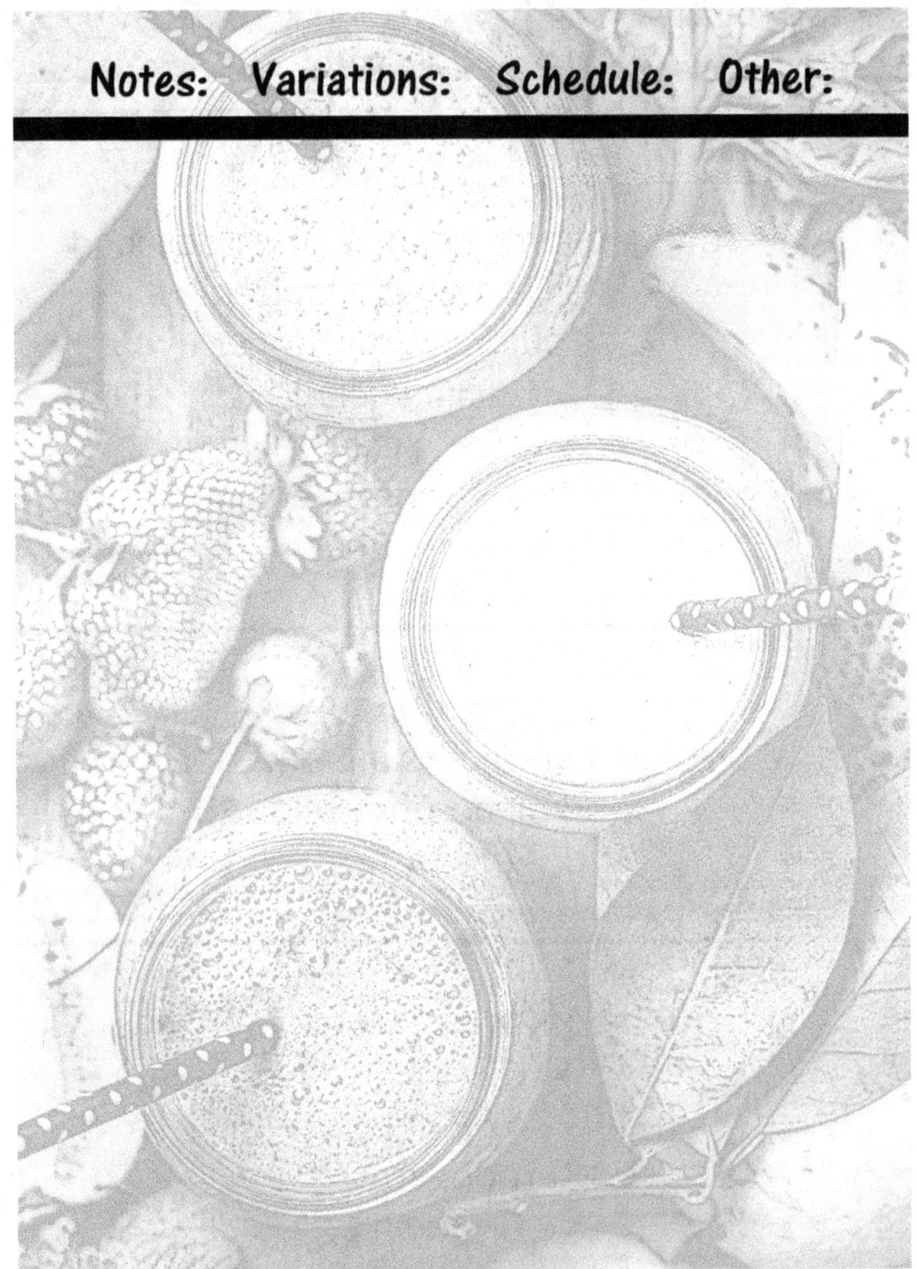

Mango Madness Smoothie

Ingredients
- 1 cup frozen mango chunks, peeled
- ½ cup frozen strawberries, unsweetened
- 1 banana, peeled
- ¼ tsp. cayenne pepper
- ½ tsp cinnamon
- 1 – 2 tsp turmeric powder
- ½ cup water
- 2 – 4 ice cubes

Directions
1. Combine ingredients in a blender. Cover and blend until smooth.
2. Serve & enjoy!

Nutritional Information (per serving)
- Calories 187
- Fat 1 g
- Carbohydrates 40 g
- Protein 1 g

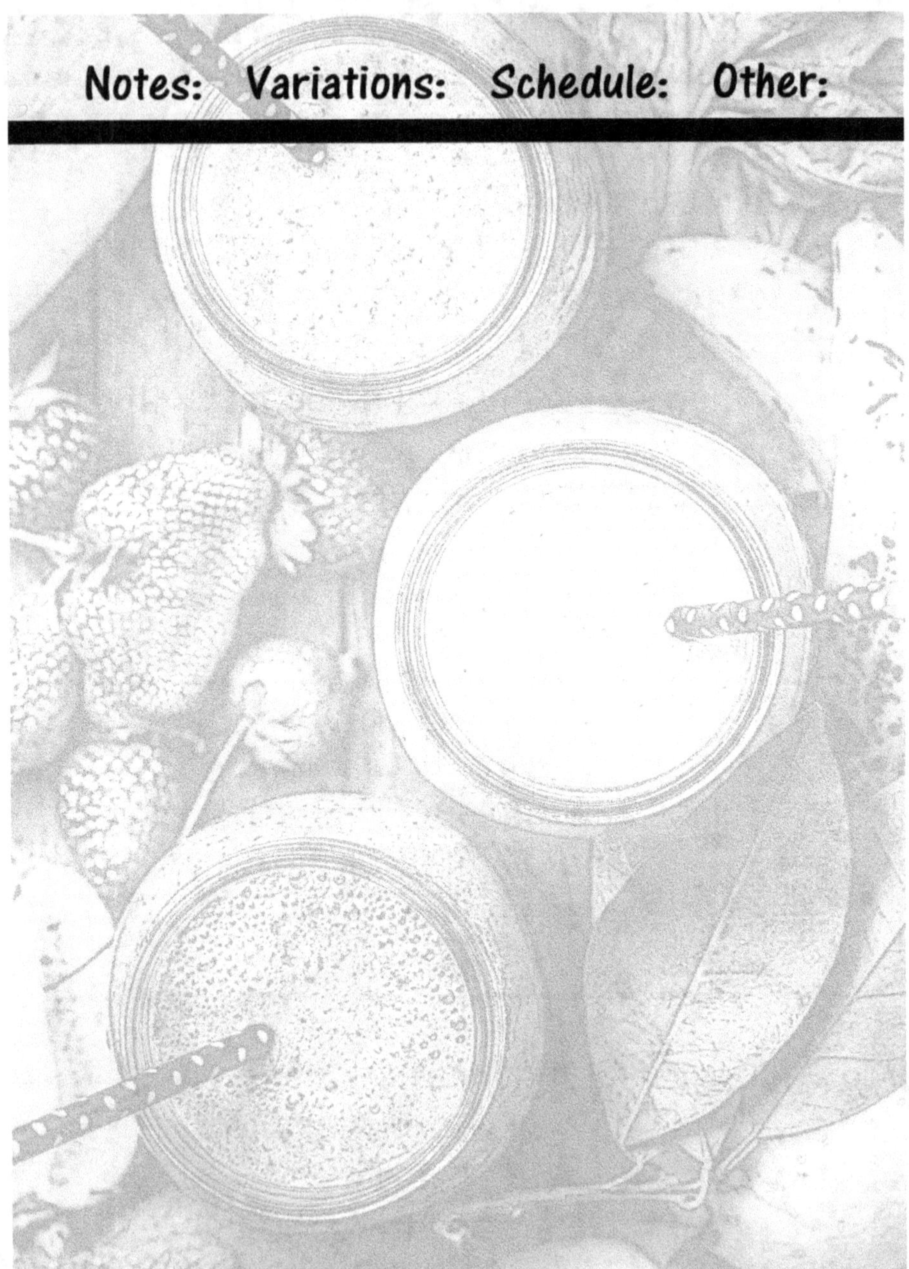

Cherry Berry Smoothie

Ingredients
- 1 cup romaine lettuce, chopped
- ½ cup dark cherries, pitted
- 1 cup blueberries
- 1/2 cup cherry juice – from concentrate
- 1 – 2 tsp turmeric powder
- 4-6 ice cubes

Directions
1. Combine ingredients in a blender. Cover and blend until smooth.
2. Serve & enjoy!

Nutritional Information (per serving)
- Calories 177
- Fat 0 g
- Carbohydrates 38 g
- Protein 1 g

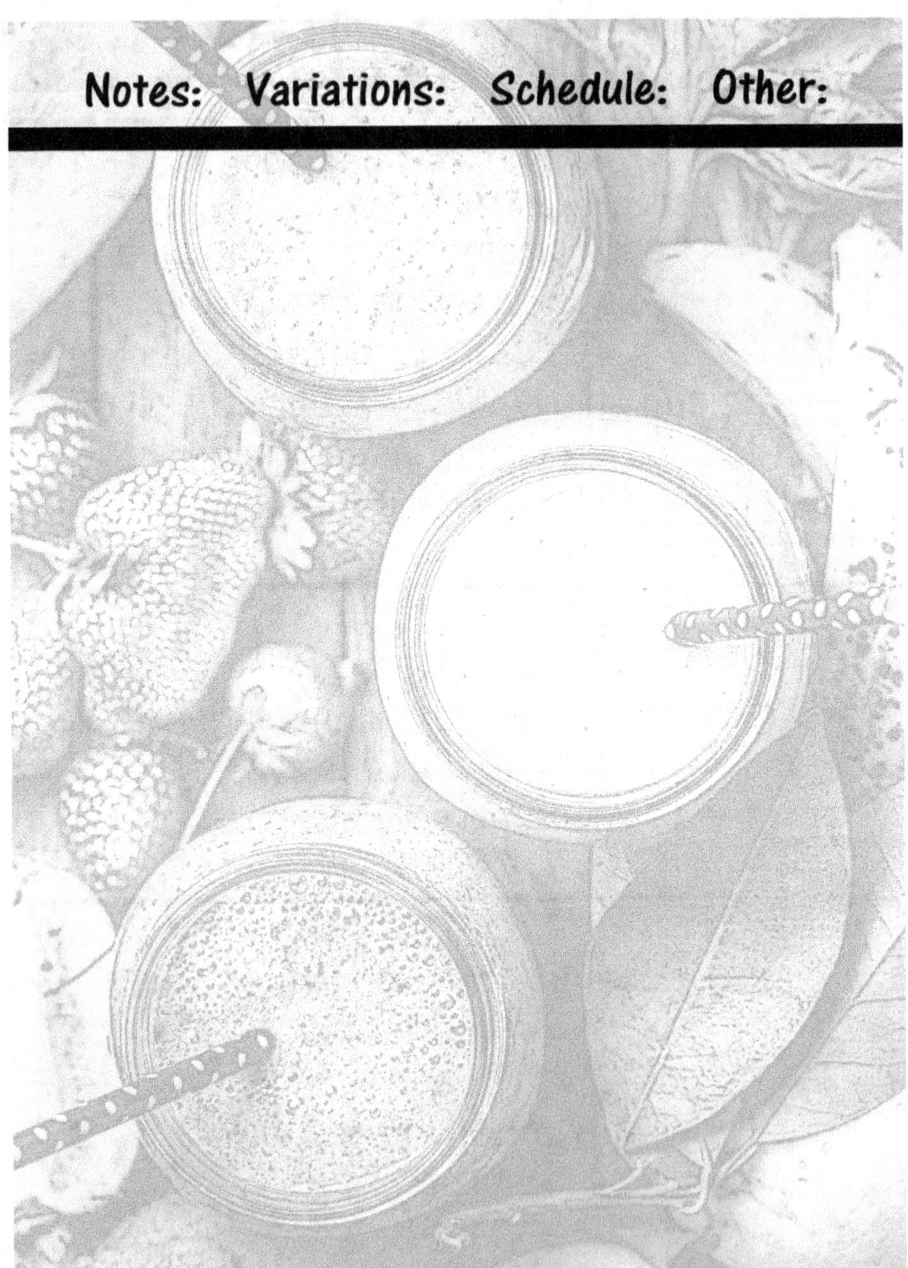

Ingredients

- ¼ cup watercress
- 1 small avocado, pitted and peeled
- 1 green apple, cored and quartered, with skin
- 1/2 cup apple cider
- 1 – 2 tsp turmeric powder
- 3-6 ice cubes

Directions

1. Combine ingredients in a blender. Cover and blend until smooth.
2. Serve & Enjoy!

Nutritional Information (per serving)

- Calories 285
- Fat 15 g
- Carbohydrates 34 g
- Protein 2 g

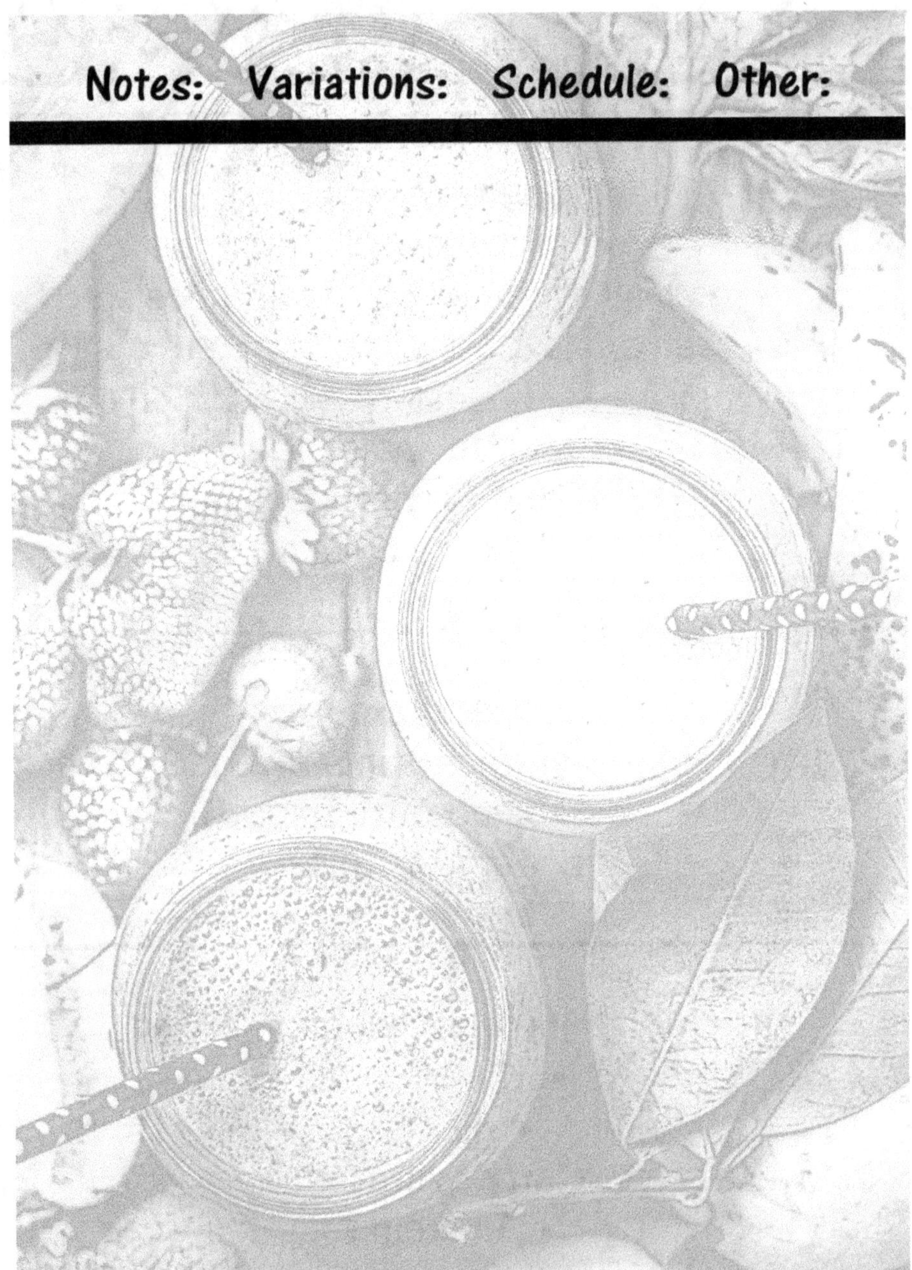

Join the free Gout & Inflammation Newsletter. Clickable links are inside of the eBook version of this book. Or, you can also email **goutinflammationinfo@gmail.com** and request the link to be sent to your email.

If you enjoyed these recipes, your reviews are always appreciated! Thank you!

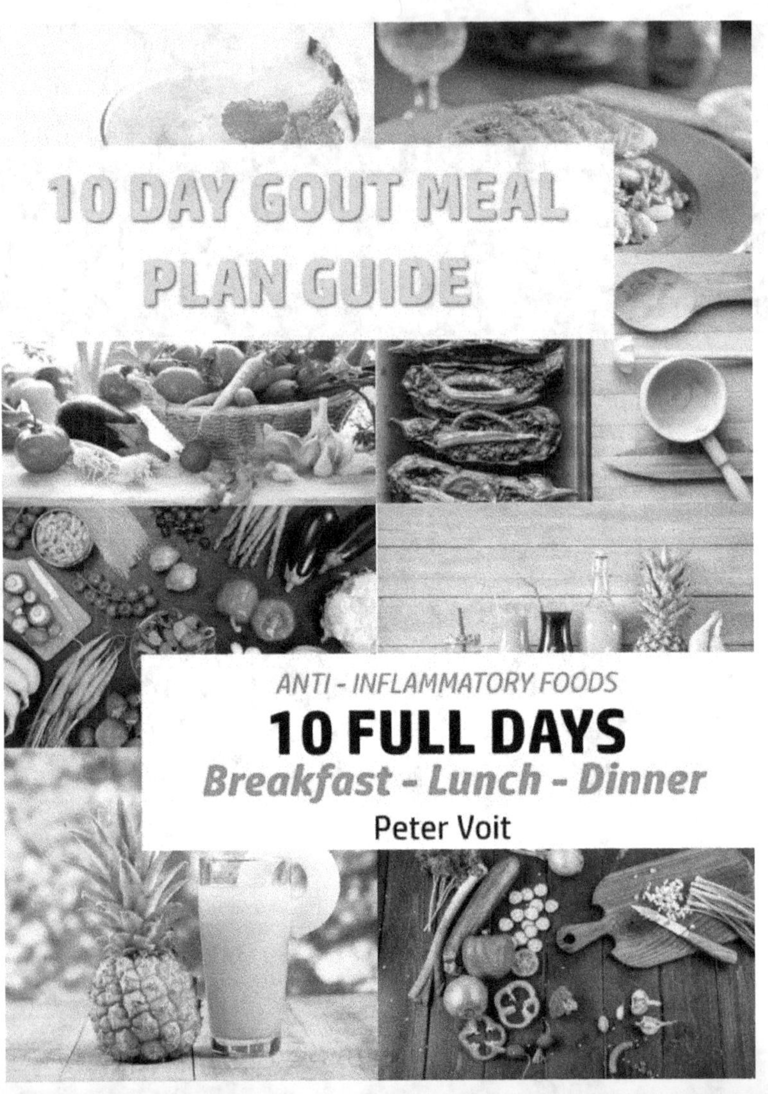

10 DAY GOUT MEAL PLAN GUIDE
ANTI - INFLAMMATORY FOODS
10 FULL DAYS
Breakfast - Lunch - Dinner
Peter Voit

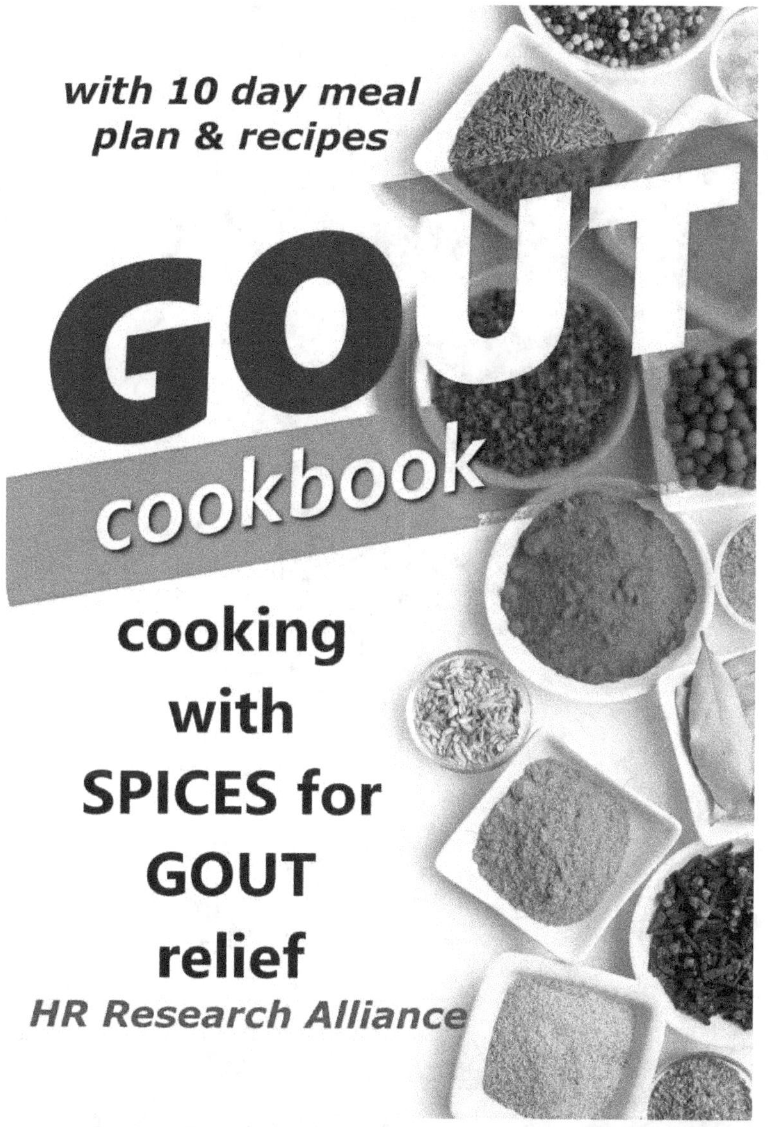

with 10 day meal plan & recipes
GOUT
cookbook
cooking
with
SPICES for
GOUT
relief
HR Research Alliance

Everything You Must Know About Gout

HR Research Alliance

Gout

The Ultimate Guide

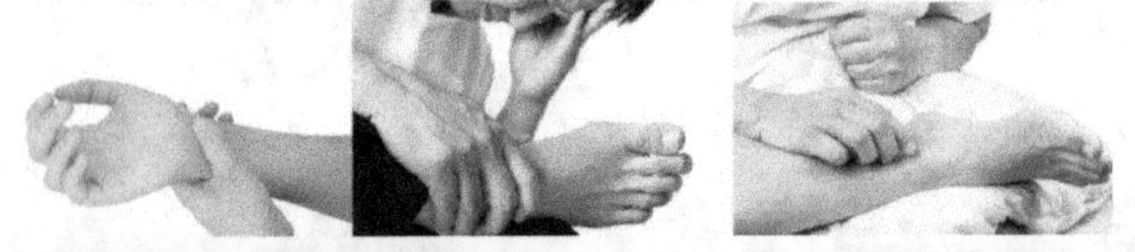

For some great information on gout, check this book out on Amazon.

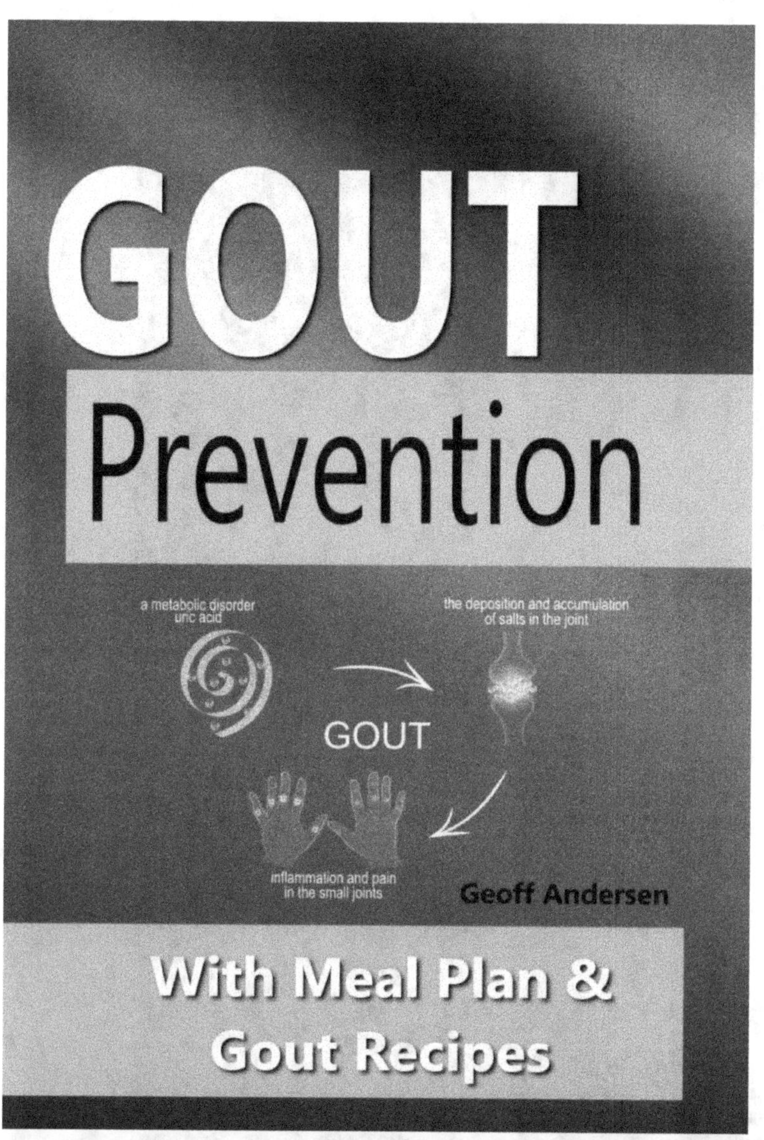

This book contains some really valuable information on gout. Look for it on Amazon.

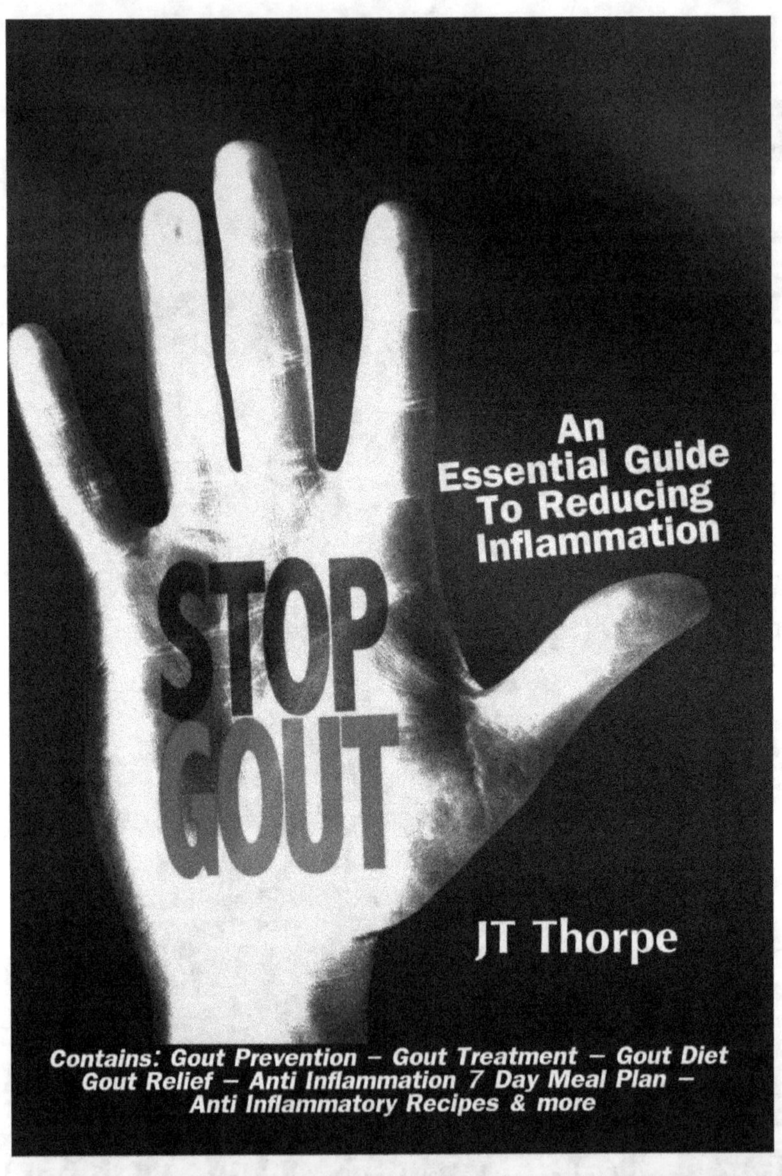

A great book on gout. Find it on Amazon.

Use these templates to create your own recipes.

Recipe:

Servings | Prep Time | Cook Time

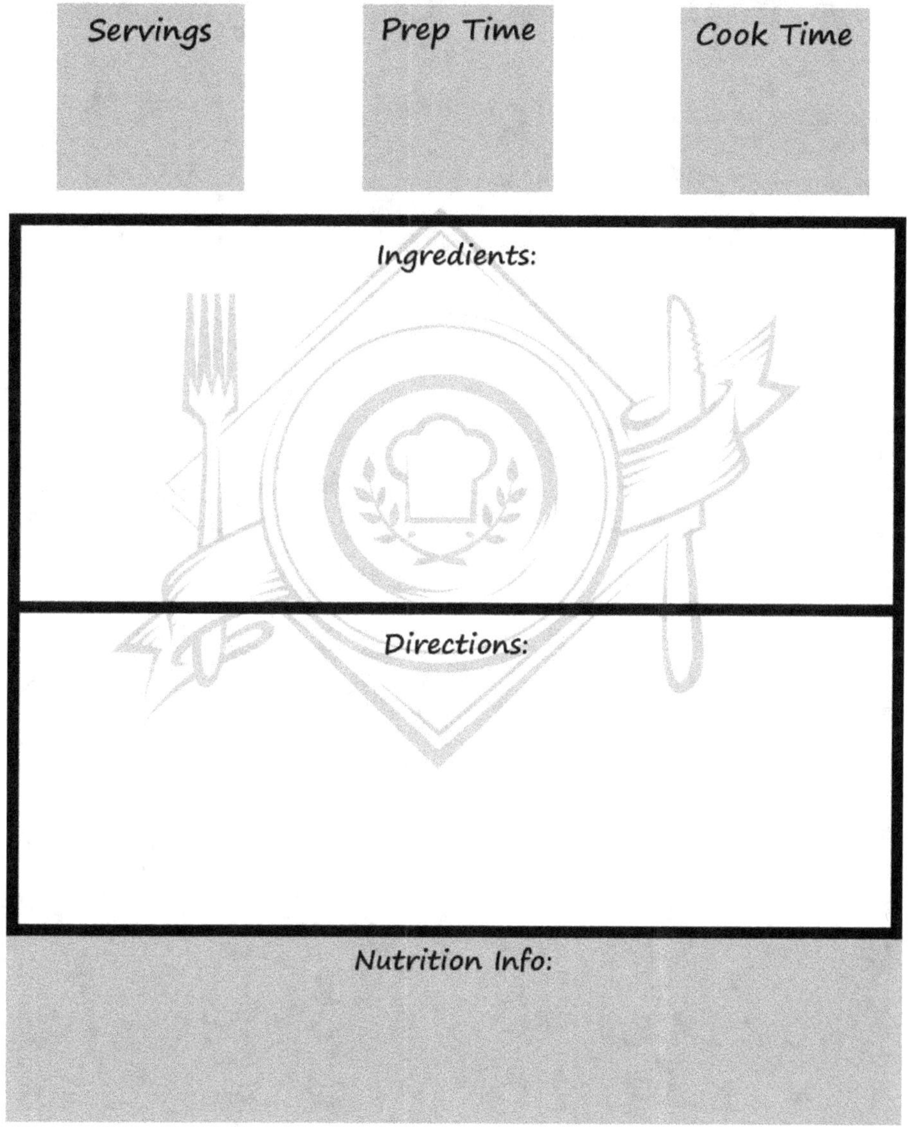

Ingredients:

Directions:

Nutrition Info:

Recipe:

Servings

Prep Time

Cook Time

Ingredients:

Directions:

Nutrition Info:

Recipe:

Servings

Prep Time

Cook Time

Ingredients:

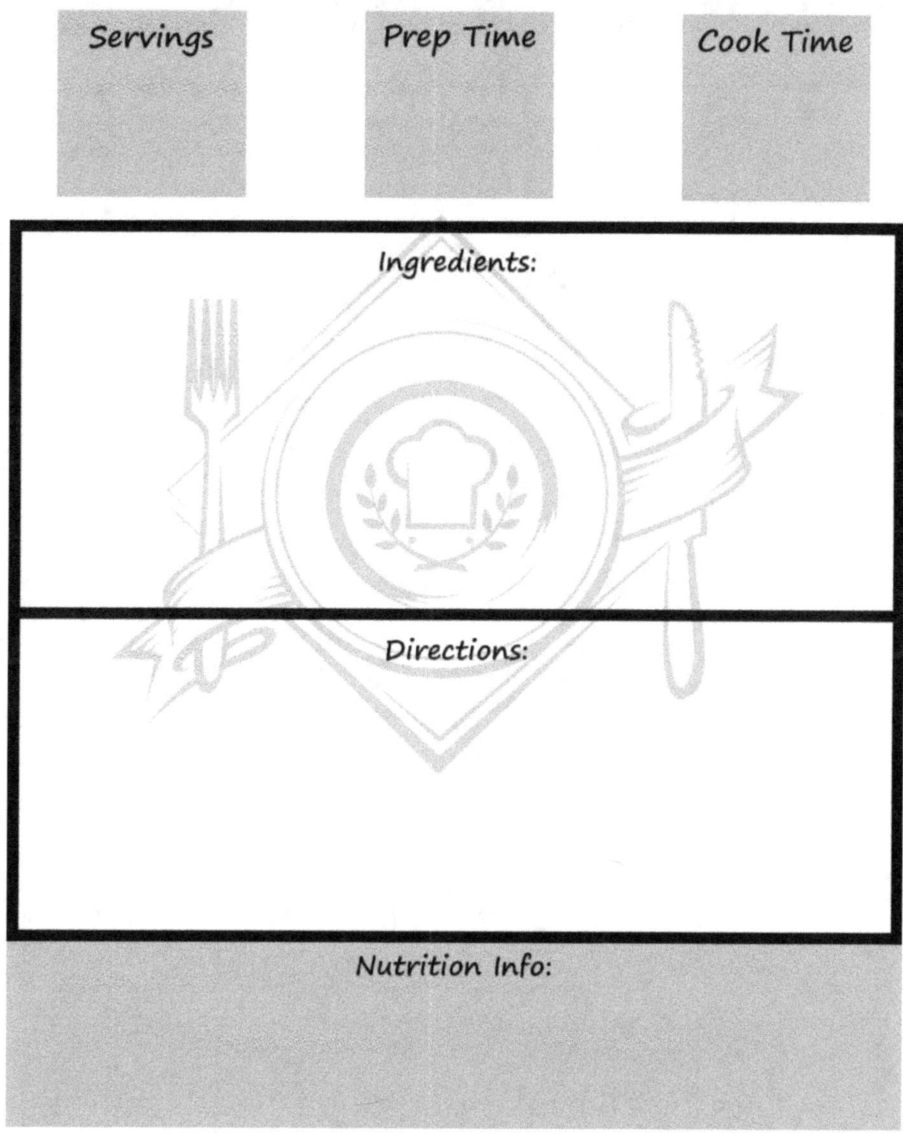

Directions:

Nutrition Info:

Recipe:

Servings

Prep Time

Cook Time

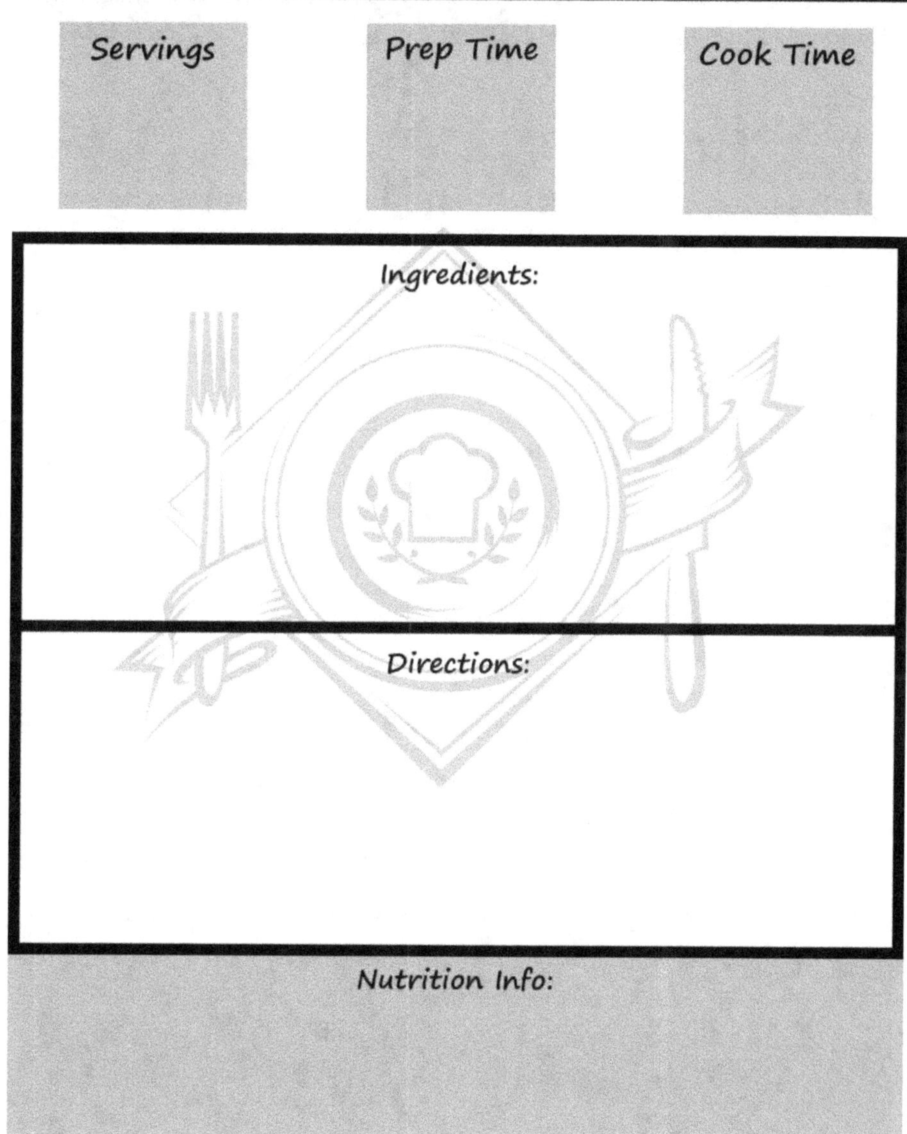

Ingredients:

Directions:

Nutrition Info:

Recipe:

Servings

Prep Time

Cook Time

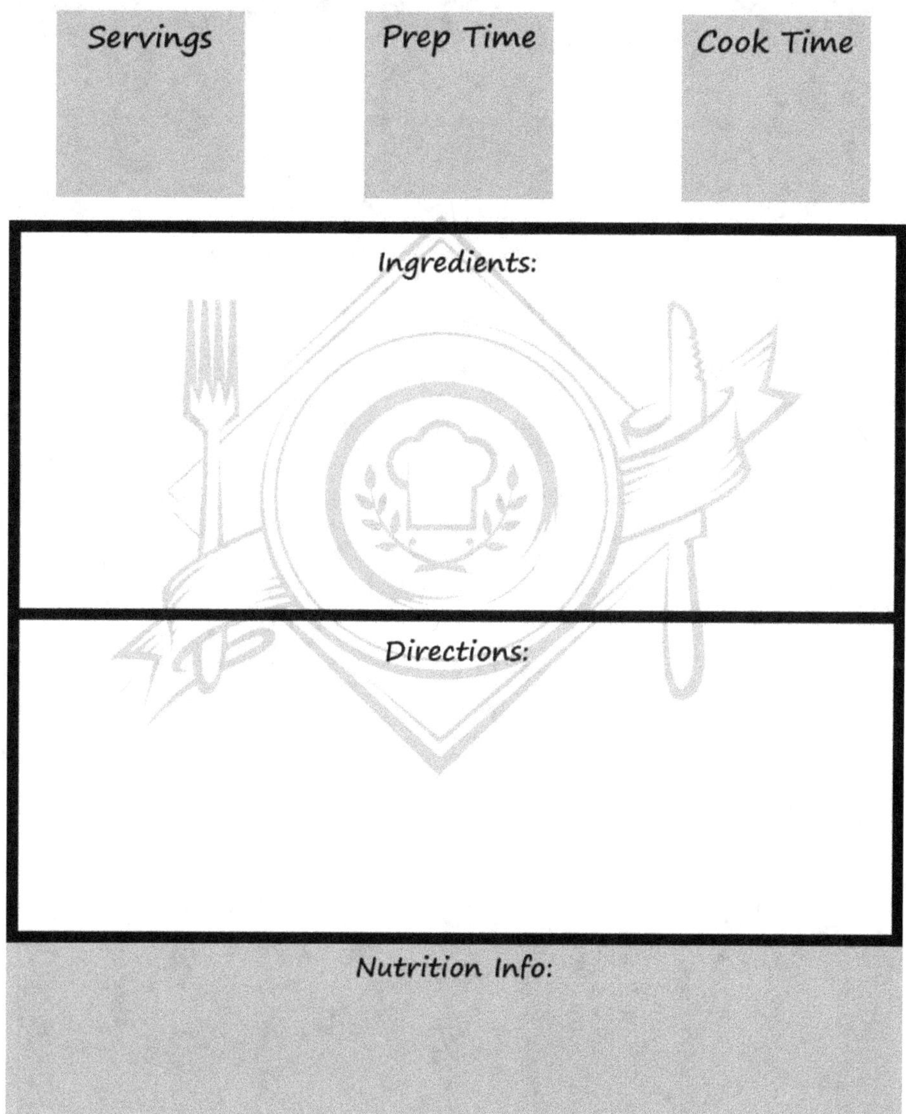

Ingredients:

Directions:

Nutrition Info:

Notes

Servings

Prep Time

Cook Time

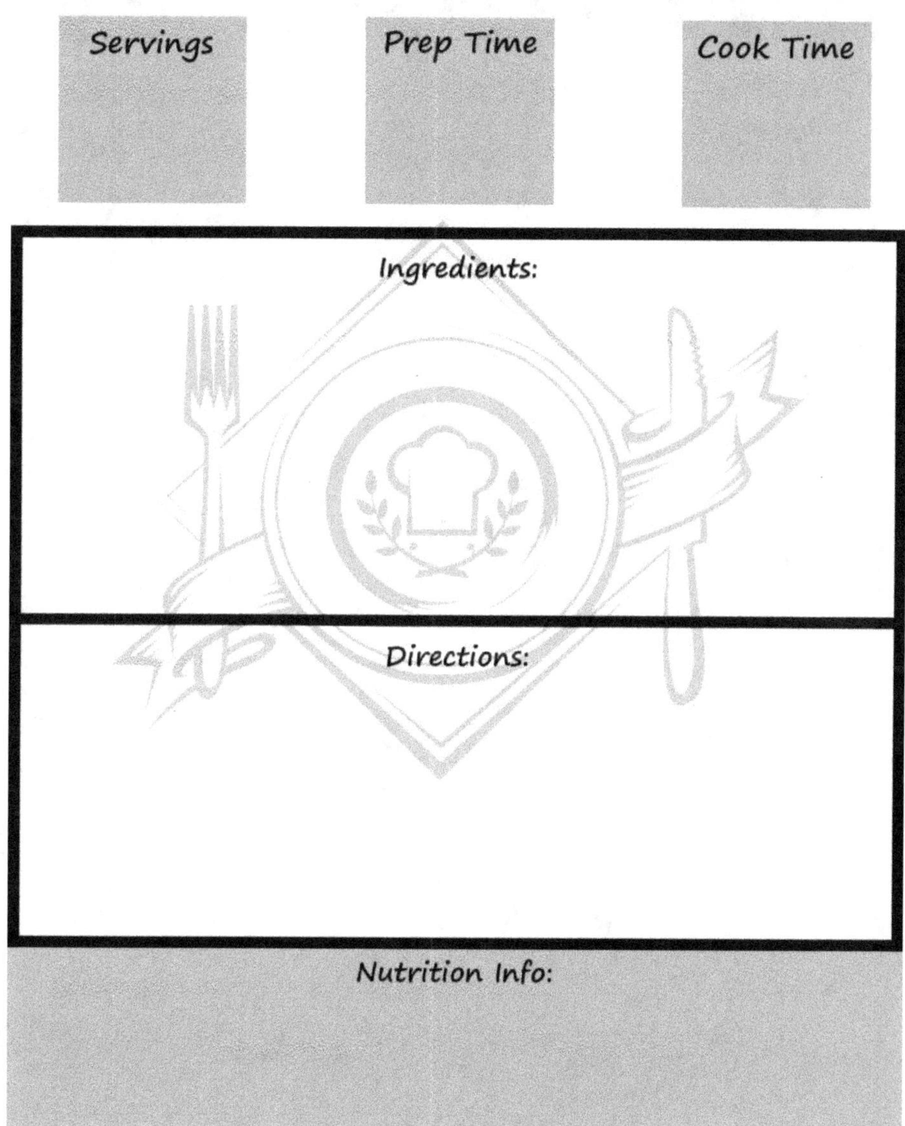

Ingredients:

Directions:

Nutrition Info:

Recipe:

Servings

Prep Time

Cook Time

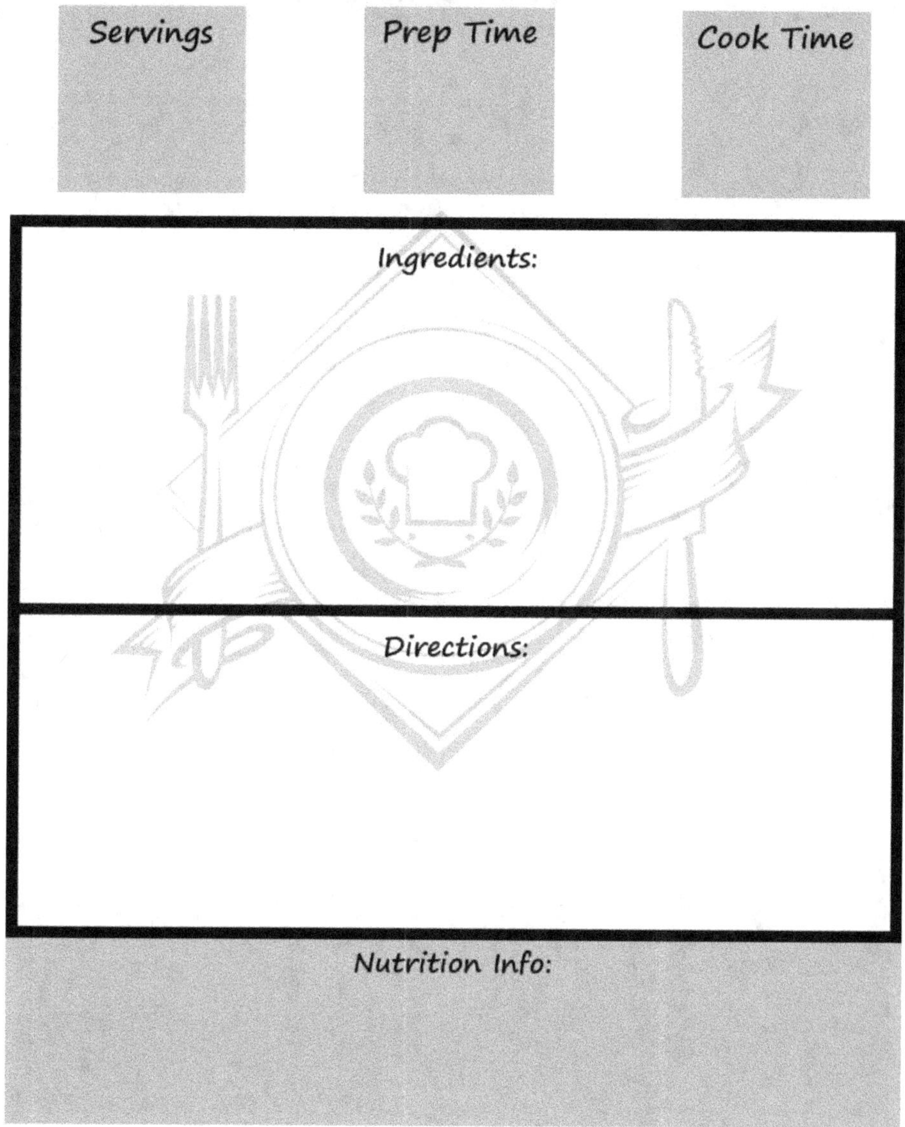

Ingredients:

Directions:

Nutrition Info:

Recipe:

| Servings | Prep Time | Cook Time |

Ingredients:

Directions:

Nutrition Info:

Recipe:

| Servings | Prep Time | Cook Time |

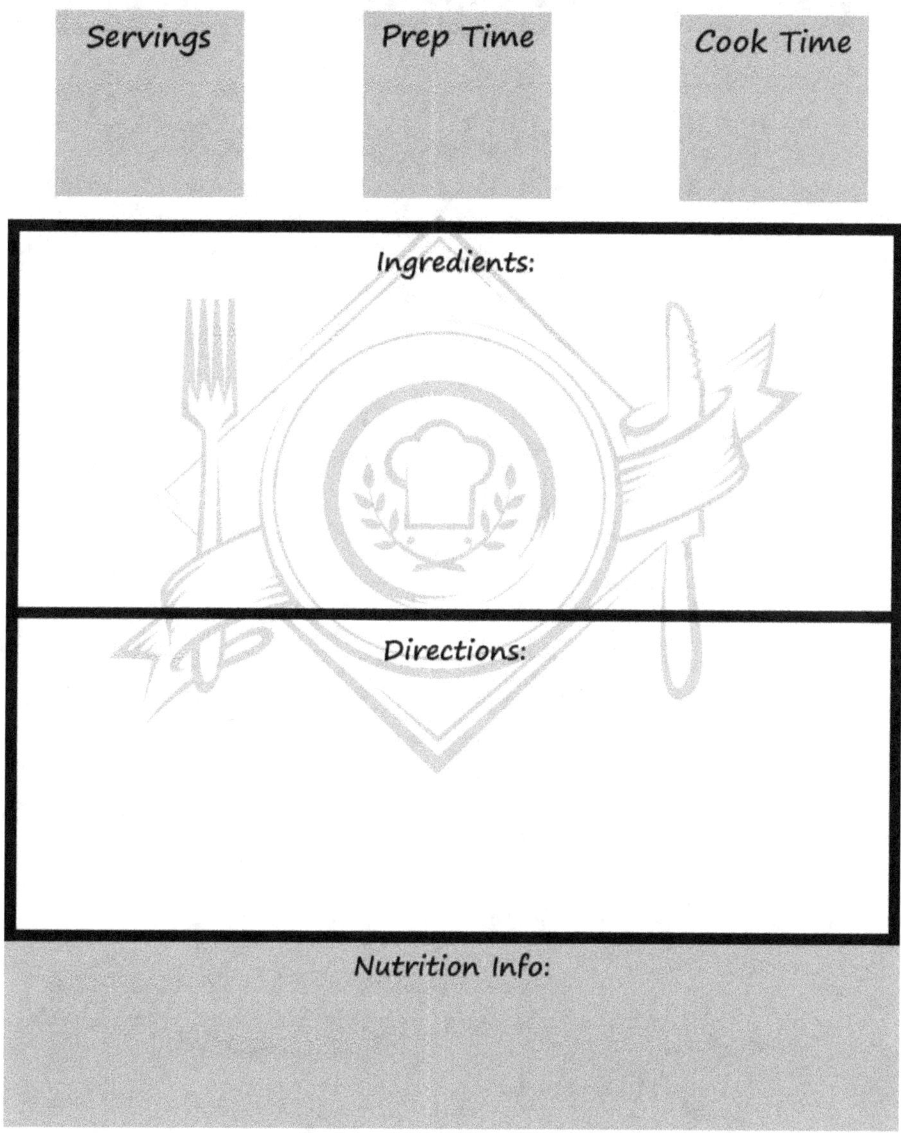

Ingredients:

Directions:

Nutrition Info:

Recipe:

| Servings | Prep Time | Cook Time |

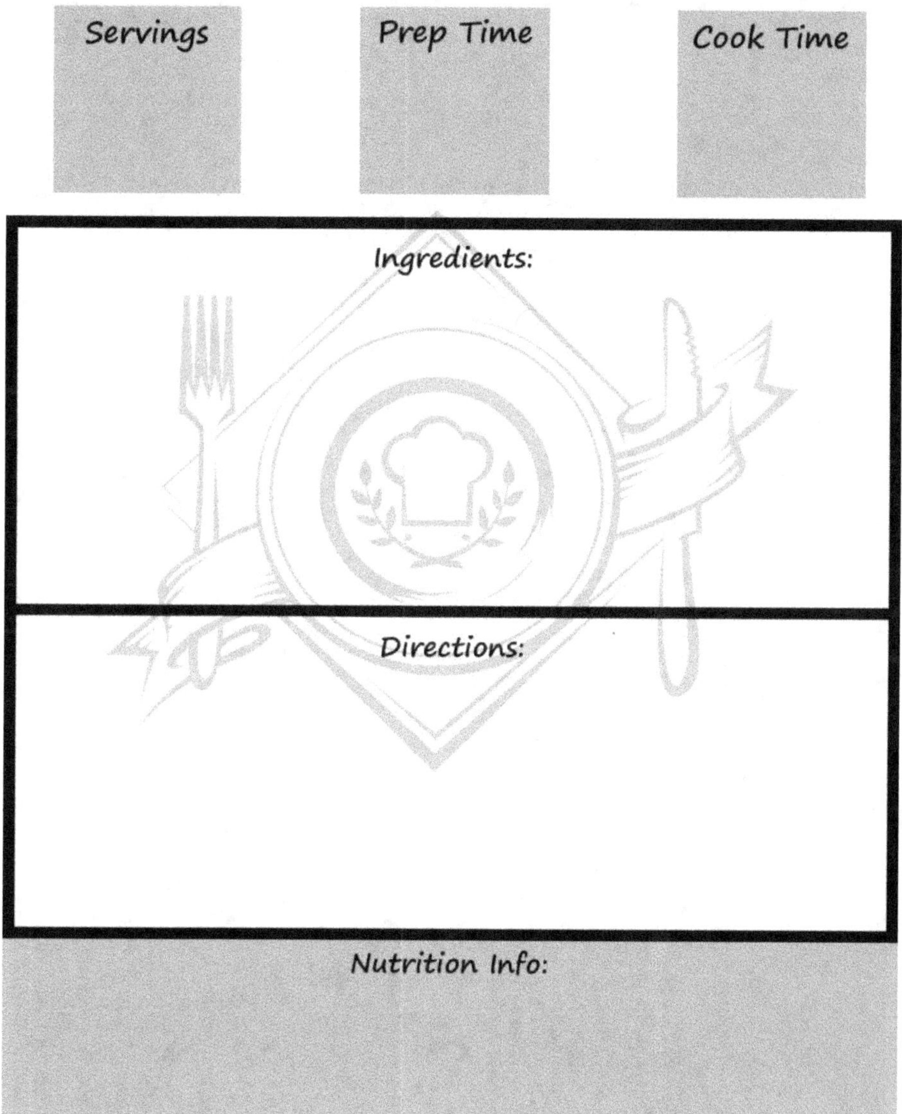

Ingredients:

Directions:

Nutrition Info:

Recipe:

Servings

Prep Time

Cook Time

Ingredients:

Directions:

Nutrition Info:

Recipe:

Servings   Prep Time   Cook Time

Ingredients:

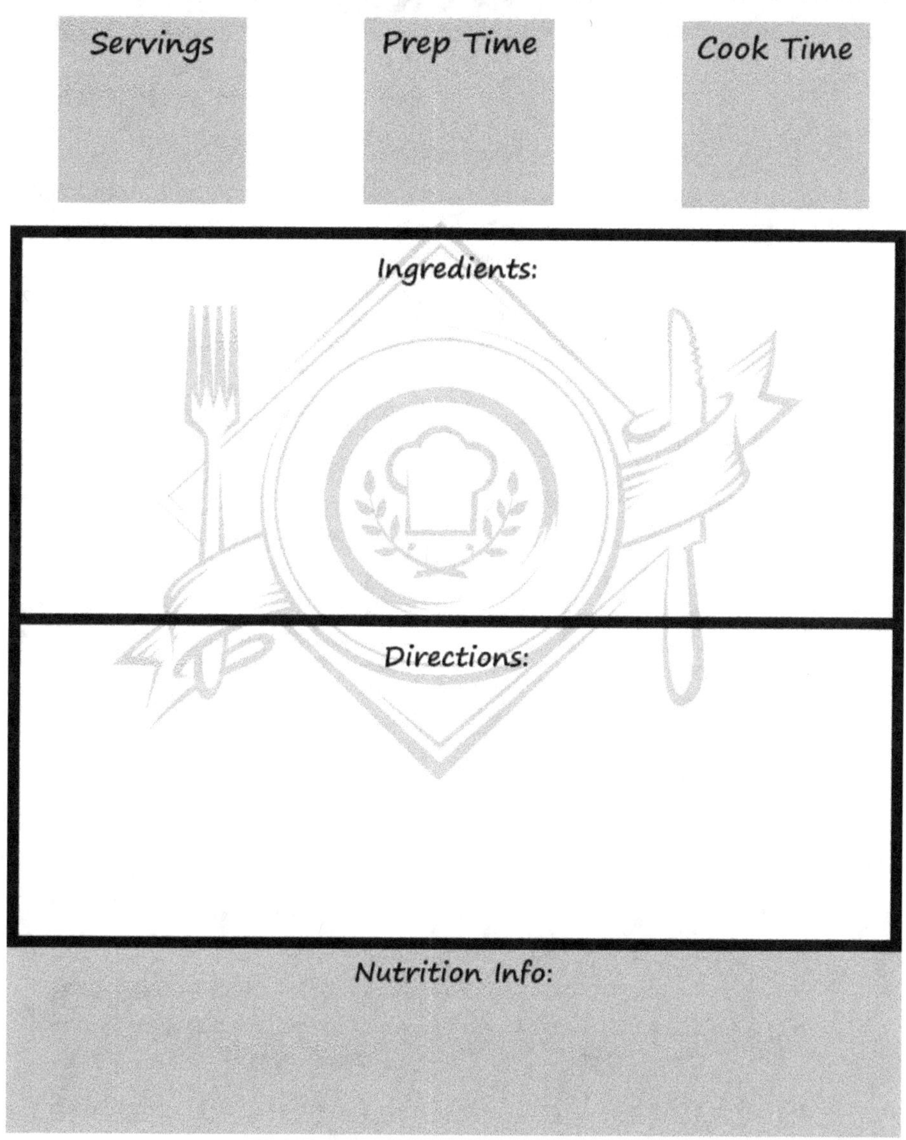

Directions:

Nutrition Info:

www.ingramcontent.com/pod-product-compliance
Lightning Source LLC
Chambersburg PA
CBHW070130260726
48658CB00001B/342